# OUTSMARTING
# DIABETES

## A Dynamic Approach for Reducing the Effects of Insulin-Dependent Diabetes

Richard S. Beaser, M.D.
Joslin Diabetes Center
Boston, Massachusetts

OUTSMARTING DIABETES
A Dynamic Approach for Reducing the Effects of Insulin-Dependent Diabetes, © 1994 by Joslin Diabetes Center

**Library of Congress Cataloging-in-Publication Data**
        Beaser, Richard S., M.D.
        Outsmarting Diabetes: A Dynamic Approach for
        Reducing the Effects of Insulin-Dependent Diabetes
                p.        cm.
            ISBN 1-56561-051-2 (pbk.) $14.95
            1. Diabetes—Treatment. 2. Insulin. 3. Insulin pumps.
        I. Title.
        RC660.B364        1994
        616.4'6206—dc20                94-11324
                                        CIP


Edited by: Donna Hoel
Cover design: Emerson, Wajdowicz Studios, Inc./NYC
Interior design: Liana Vaiciulis Raudys


10 9 8 7 6 5 4 3 2 1

Published by: CHRONIMED Publishing
P.O. Box 47945
Minneapolis, MN  55447-9727

# Table of Contents

A book of this nature cannot be written without the assistance and support of others. Intensive diabetes therapy and, of course, diabetes treatment in general is a team effort. There are many members of the "team" who I would like to acknowledge.

Donna Richardson, R.N., C.D.E., past director of patient education, and Laurinda Poirier, R.N., C.D.E., the director of clinical and educational services at the Joslin Diabetes Center, were most supportive of this effort with time, advice, and moral support. Debra Conboy, R.N., C.D.E., our diabetes nurse educator who specializes in intensive diabetes therapy, as well as Susan Crowell, R.N., C.D.E., the head DCCT research nurse at the Joslin Diabetes Center site, provided tremendous amounts of insight and expertise. Carrie Stewart, R.N., M.S., C.D.E., Joslin DCCT nurse, also helped.

I would also like to acknowledge my colleagues with whom I worked as investigators as part of the DCCT team at Joslin: Alan Jacobson, M.D., Om Ganda, M.D., James Rosenzweig, M.D., and Joseph Wolfsdorf, M.D., and our study ophthalmologist, George Sharuk, M.D.

Joan Hill, R.D., C.D.E., Joslin's director of nutrition services, Beverly Halford, R.D., C.D.E., dietitian with the DCCT at the Joslin site, and Melinda Maryniuk, R.D., C.D.E., of Joslin's Affiliated Centers Program contributed their expertise to the sections on nutrition. In general, all members of the Joslin staff of Diabetes Nurse Educators and Registered Dietitians, working with our patients, either directly or indirectly provided assistance in the preparation of this book.

Joy Kistler, M.S., C.D.E., Joslin's exercise physiologist, provided input on the exercise section. Barbara Anderson, Ph.D., C.D.E., from our mental health section assisted with preparation of the chapter on the psychological impact of intensive therapy. Additional assistance and support were provided by Cynthia Pasquarella, R.N., B.S.N., C.D.E., our pediatric diabetes nurse educator. Julie Rafferty, director of communications, Thomas McCullough, public information manager, and Ray Moloney, director of publications at Joslin, also helped by coordinating efforts to get everybody's comments on the draft of this book incorporated into the final text. In addition, invaluable secretarial assistance was provided by Noreen Carson and Trisha Naughton.

Finally, I want to acknowledge the role of the 1,441 patients who volunteered for the Diabetes Control and Complications Trial (DCCT). While intensive diabetes therapy was being used before and during this study, it was this trial that proved, finally, that the effort involved in this treatment is worth it. These 1,441 people made this study possible—and this book necessary!

# Can Diabetes Complications Be Prevented?

- What do we mean by control?

- Why is the DCCT study important?

- What does "intensive" mean?

- How can all this help you?

## What does "control" mean?

If there's a health catchword for the '90s, it has to be *control*. In managing your diabetes, you hear the word probably more often than you would like. It means keeping your blood glucose levels as near to those of a person without diabetes as you possibly can. But will carefully controlling your blood glucose reduce your risks for eye problems, nerve degeneration, kidney failure, heart disease, or strokes?

Since the discovery of insulin, physicians and researchers have been guessing about the role control plays in reducing complications. Now we have some answers. Early in 1993, a major study called the Diabetes Control and Complications Trial, or DCCT, was stopped a full year early because of its dramatic and conclusive findings—that control matters. The Joslin Diabetes Center was one of the 29 centers participating in this study.

## What is the DCCT?

The DCCT was started in the early 1980s to test the question: "Will normalization or near normalization of blood glucose levels in people with diabetes help to delay or prevent diabetes complications?" In addition, the study looked at whether it is practical and safe to maintain blood glucose levels in the normal or near-normal range in people with diabetes.

This long-term, multicenter study, sponsored by the National Institutes of Health (NIH), involved 1,441 volunteers aged 13 to 39, with type I, insulin-dependent diabetes. Half the volunteers used what has been known as "conventional" diabetes management: They took one or two injections of insulin each day, monitored their blood glucose or urine once a day, were given dietary education, and saw their physicians and diabetes health care teams four times a year.

The other half of the patients used what is commonly called "intensive" therapy. This involved three or more injections each day or use of an insulin pump. Insulin was adjusted on the basis of four or more daily blood glucose tests. This group also had intensive diabetes education and dietary, exercise, and psychological counseling. They saw their physicians and diabetes health care teams every month.

Both groups were watched closely for signs of eye, nerve, and kidney disease. And the differences between the two groups was stunning.

## The outcomes

With intensive therapy, the incidence of eye complications was reduced by as much as 76 percent. Kidney complications were reduced by up to 56 percent, and nerve problems by up to 60 percent. The study wasn't long enough to assess the heart and stroke risks, but researchers believe there is good evidence that careful "physiologic" control improves these risks also. By physiologic, we mean control that is as close as possible to what the nondiabetic body would do.

A measurement called the *glycosylated hemoglobin test* showed that the lower the amount of glucose in the blood for an extended period of time, the lower the risk for long-term complications.

## What's the downside?

The main problem with intensive diabetes therapy is the high risk of insulin reactions. Even though the people who used the intensive program checked their blood four or more times a day, they had three times more severe low blood sugar reactions than the conventional treatment group. (By severe, we mean reactions requiring assistance from someone or emergency room visits.)

People using the intensive plan also gained weight. After five years, most were about 10 pounds heavier than matched partners using conventional treatment. This could be because the body uses calories more efficiently when insulin levels are kept closer to a nondiabetic level. Or it could be that increased flexibility in using insulin encourages people to eat more of the things they formerly avoided.

Another disadvantage is that the intensive approach is more expensive than conventional therapy—at least in the short run. However, once the cost of complications is added, intensive therapy seems to be a much better investment.

With proper training and follow-up, working together with your physician, dietitian, and nurse educator, you should be able to reduce significantly the risk of severe hypoglycemia and weight gain.

## How intensive is intensive?

There are no magic numbers for glucose or for glycosylated hemoglobin. But the DCCT study showed that the closer to normal, nondiabetic levels, the better. Therefore, any improvement in your control, regardless of how high you are at the start and how much you are able to improve it, will be of benefit to you.

In the DCCT study, the goals were:

- Fasting and premeal blood glucose levels of 70
  to 120 mg/dl
- After-meal levels of less than 180 mg
- 3 A.M. levels of more than 65 mg
- Glycosylated hemoglobin as close to normal
  as possible (For the people in the DCCT study,
  this was about 6.05 percent, but the numbers vary
  depending on laboratory standards.)

## What does this mean for you?

Every step you take toward better diabetes control can mean fewer problems in the future. Of course, there are no guarantees. But if you're looking at the facts, intensive therapy is the best approach for many people—both those with type I and perhaps those with type II on insulin. It's a tough choice, though, and you need to make a serious commitment to change many aspects of your life.

If you have newly diagnosed diabetes, you may not need to start with an intensive plan. Also, older people who are at risk of harm from falls or other medical problems if they have severe insulin reactions and others who want to avoid reactions won't want to set their sights on extremely rigid control. But there may well be a middle ground that would be beneficial, and working together with your health care team, you can find the proper balance that is right for you.

## How will this book help?

This book will give you information about intensified conventional and truly intensive approaches to diabetes management—both through multiple injection plans and through insulin pump programs. It will explain how good physiologic control works and what to expect as you move toward it. The goal is to give you information to help you work with your health care team to improve your own diabetes management.

Throughout this book, we provide information on how to start various types of intensive and intensified diabetes therapy programs. In some cases, we will list blood glucose goals that are somewhat less stringent than those targeted by the DCCT guidelines listed above. We do this intentionally. Our goal is to allow you to safely start your intensive program. Ultimately, you and your health care team may wish to aim for these DCCT-recommended goals, should they be deemed safely achievable by you.

The DCCT study has shown that any and all improvements in diabetes control can reduce your risk for complications. You need to check with your health care team about what plan would work best to get you moving in the right direction.

# Chapter One

# What Is Intensive Management?

What's this section about?

■ Why is this possible now?

■ What's conventional, conventional intensified, and true intensive management?

■ How much control do you need?

■ Why should you try this?

You may be interested in intensive therapy for a variety of reasons, each one legitimate and proper if you or someone close to you has diabetes. Some of your reasons might include the following:

- You've heard of intensive therapy and want to know more about it.
- You hope intensive therapy may normalize your blood glucose patterns and help you feel better.
- You believe intensive therapy may help prevent complications.
- You've had unsatisfactory control with conventional insulin therapy.
- Your conventional therapy leaves severe blood glucose fluctuations, both disruptive and dangerous.
- You feel that intensive insulin therapy is the best way to control your diabetes in spite of your unpredictable or hectic lifestyle.
- You are considering getting pregnant in the near future.

Whatever your reasons, intensive insulin therapy allows and requires *you,* with guidance from your health team, to take charge of your diabetes. Intensive therapy demands more awareness on your part, but offers much closer control of your blood glucose levels through careful attention to diet, exercise, and other factors known to affect diabetes.

## Why is this treatment available now?

Intensive treatment is possible now because of two improvements in diabetes care: the glycohemoglobin test (also called glycosylated hemoglobin, hemoglobin $A_1c$, or $HbA_1c$), which measures overall diabetes control, and self-monitoring of blood glucose, which allows frequent assessment of blood glucose levels and adjustment to try to correct them. These tools are also used for conventional therapy.

## What is glycohemoglobin?

As glucose circulates in the blood, it attaches itself to proteins. This happens in everyone, regardless of whether diabetes is present. For people with higher blood glucose levels, though, more proteins are carrying glucose because there is more glucose in the blood.

Hemoglobin is a red blood cell protein that carries oxygen from the lungs to the rest of the body. Hemoglobin with glucose attached to it is called glycohemoglobin, glycosylated hemoglobin, or hemoglobin $A_1c$. When diabetes isn't present, about 3 to 6 percent of cells carry glucose. With diabetes the percentage can be much higher.

The glycohemoglobin test, which is done at a clinic or laboratory, shows the average blood glucose over about three months—the normal life of a red blood cell. The test is seldom affected by an occasional high or low glucose level or even several days of poor control.

Glycohemoglobin measurements provide good information about whether blood glucose control is better than, or not as good as, daily monitoring shows. The test is an excellent tool for helping you set goals. Ask your diabetes team what your glycohemoglobin levels are and exactly what the numbers mean. (Test results vary, depending on how they're done.)

So there is no misunderstanding, we need to say again that conventional therapy is appropriate for people who can maintain control using it. The intensive approach offers the possibility of even better control for those who want and need closer self-monitoring.

While you read this manual, keep in mind the fundamentals of diabetes—why it occurs, how it is treated conventionally with insulin, what the dangers and possible complications are.*

## How do the approaches differ?

As you read about intensive therapy, ask your doctor or health team for details on how it can help *you*. You're the one in charge with this type of treatment, but you'll need close contact with the professionals, especially at first.

*Conventional therapy* uses the same insulin dose (fixed dose) each day. Some people with type I diabetes and many with type II diabetes needing insulin can be successfully treated with the conventional approach. In contrast, *intensive therapy* uses either multiple daily injections (MDI) of insulin or an infusion pump that provides a continuous subcutaneous (under the skin) insulin infusion. The goal of this type of therapy is to reach and maintain a specific range for blood glucose.

Some people may choose a middle ground—*intensified conventional therapy*—which combines the simpler treatment approach of conventional therapy with some of the flexibility of the more intensive approach.

With the *intensive or intensified conventional* programs, premeal insulin doses are adjusted according to blood glucose measurements taken at the time. You also can adjust to compensate for variations in diet, exercise, and other factors that affect blood glucose levels.

To help determine the proper doses, people frequently use a sliding scale or *algorithm*, which is an insulin dose adjustment plan. They test

---

* If you do not have a good understanding of diabetes, ask your health care team for material or contact the Joslin Diabetes Center, (617) 732-2415, for information on how to order materials on the fundamentals of diabetes.

their blood glucose at dose time and consult their algorithm for the correct insulin dose.

## What each approach assumes

*Conventional fixed-dose* therapy assumes that, as long as food consumption, activity, and timing are relatively consistent, insulin requirements will be the same each day. By contrast, *intensive therapy* assumes that insulin needs vary from day to day. These variations occur because blood glucose levels are affected by many factors.

In fact, insulin requirements *do* vary from day to day, and the variation has a greater effect on blood sugar control in some people than others.

You may choose to intensify your therapy because daily variations in your insulin requirements are a concern for you. To use the more intensive approach, you must make more frequent and exact measurements of blood glucose levels, pay more attention to variations in factors that affect your diabetes, and use a more systematic scheme to compensate for these variations.

Intensive diabetes therapy is not so much a different treatment as it is a more intensive way of using conventional treatments. There are no dividing lines among the approaches. Rather, they represent different degrees of intensity.

## Understanding your choices

Conventional therapy is the simplest approach. Intensified conventional therapy requires more care in monitoring and understanding what is affecting your blood glucose. Finally, the intensive approach requires a good bit more attention to the details of diabetes management. Choosing the degree of intensity that is right for you requires thoughtful discussion with your health care team.

| Conventional therapy | Conventional intensified therapy | True intensive therapy |
|---|---|---|
| Uses fixed-dose insulin that assumes eating and exercise are roughly the same each day | Involves more testing and more adjustments of insulin for meals and exercise | Involves more testing and multiple daily injections or use of an insulin pump |

## Evolution of intensive therapy

In the early years of insulin therapy, all insulins were similar to the short-acting insulin (regular) we use today. Patients often gave themselves four to six daily injections. With the development of the longer-acting insulins (PZI, NPH, lente, and ultralente), the number of daily injections could be reduced while successfully and safely eliminating the symptoms of high blood glucose.

Diabetes control was based on an office blood glucose measurement, and the only self-monitoring was urine testing. Little was known about the normal dynamics of insulin secretion and action. Many people were satisfied that, by eliminating high blood glucose symptoms with good office blood test results, these longer-acting insulins provided adequate blood glucose control.

However, a number of physicians, including those at the Joslin Clinic, believed elimination of symptoms was not enough. They reasoned that the closer the blood glucose levels were to "normal," the better off the individual would be. They also believed an insulin replacement program that mimicked normal insulin secretion would be more comfortable and would help prevent potential long-term complications. The result was the "intensive therapy" of that time— use of more than one daily insulin injection.

The most common program was the **split-mix:** regular plus NPH or lente insulin given in the morning and again before supper. Perhaps this was not intensive by today's standards, but it seemed radically aggressive then!

Characteristics of normal pancreatic insulin secretion now are more clearly understood. The pancreas constantly secretes insulin into the blood, so a minimum amount is present at all times. This is known as the *"basal" insulin level.*

The pancreas also secretes additional insulin in response to the food we eat, which helps us process incoming carbohydrates and other nutrients (Figure 1). One daily injection of intermediate insulin, peaking 8 to 12 hours after injection, does not effectively reproduce this natural pattern (Figure 2).

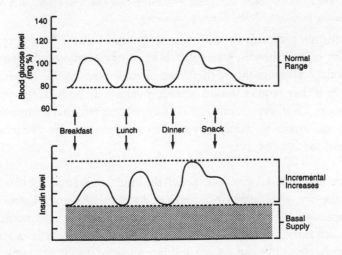

*Figure 1.* Blood glucose and insulin patterns in a person who does not have diabetes.

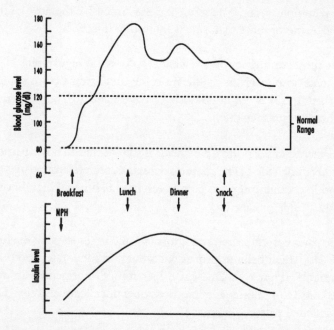

***Figure 2.*** *Blood glucose levels in a person with type I diabetes treated with one morning injection of NPH (intermediate-acting) insulin.*

Split-mix programs are still commonly used today. Many people with type I diabetes, especially those newly diagnosed, may still produce some insulin of their own. People with type II diabetes, even if they require insulin injections, also may be making some insulin. Thus, the conventional treatment program that mimics the normal insulin secretion may still be considered an effective treatment for these people.

The *classic split-mix* schedule spreads the insulin effect over the course of the day, with peaks close to times that food is eaten (Figure 3). Variations include giving the second injection as intermediate insulin alone at bedtime, or splitting the second injection to give regular insulin before supper and intermediate insulin at bedtime.

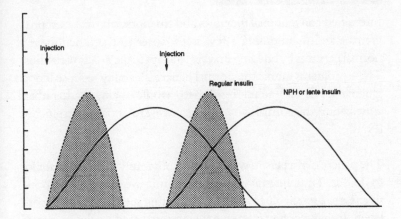

*Figure 3*. *The effect of a "split-mix" insulin program to treat type I diabetes: regular and intermediate insulin before breakfast and before supper.*

Both approaches, with the two or three daily injections, supply some insulin to the blood at all times, similar to the basal insulin of the normal pancreas.

The basis of any of these fixed-dose programs is *anticipation*. A dose of insulin is given in anticipation of the insulin needs over the next six to 12 hours. For this assumption to be correct, all factors affecting blood glucose levels must be predictable and similar, day in and day out. Eating habits, activity levels, general health, and levels of stress must be regular and predictable.

Some people *can* live their lives with enough predictability to achieve good to excellent glucose control through such a program. Many have probably retained some capacity to secrete some insulin. For those who have not, success often depends on rigid adherence to schedule and diet.

### How intensive therapies work

Intensified conventional therapies and true intensive diabetes programs take insulin dosing a few steps closer to the function of a normal pancreas by building in ways to adapt to life's daily variations. These programs mimic the normal pancreas's ability to sense blood glucose levels and adjust insulin to handle them. Rather than anticipating, the normal pancreas is *responsive* to actual blood glucose levels.

The pancreas of a person with diabetes obviously has lost the ability to do this. Thus, intensive programs mimic the pancreas's responsiveness to present glucose level by targeting specific blood glucose levels. Insulin doses in intensive therapy are based on the *anticipated* needs to reach a blood glucose goal and are *responsive* to the present glucose level.

### How good must control be?

For many years, it was not known just how good diabetes control needed to be. While many health care providers believed that fair to poor levels of control increased your chances of developing complications, the degree to which normal patterns needed to be mimicked was open to much speculation.

Now the DCCT study has given us some answers. The investigators officially concluded that "The majority of people with type I diabetes should be treated with intensive therapy with the expectation that their long-term outcome will be measurably improved."

In addition, the relationship between glycohemoglobin and complications leads to the implied conclusion that the lower the glycohemoglobin you can safely achieve, the better the chance of minimizing diabetes complications. So, for those people not choosing intensive therapy, any changes that improve diabetes control can help long-term prospects for better health.

While practical considerations may prevent some people with type I diabetes from choosing intensive therapy, for many people, particularly many of you reading this book, it may be a realistic goal.

## Who should use intensive therapy?

Not everyone can or wants to work with an intensive plan. Some people with type I diabetes who follow a  conventional insulin regimen can achieve acceptable control. If you have newly diagnosed type I diabetes, you probably should not start off with intensive therapy (unless there are special circumstances) until you understand and can manage well using conventional therapy. However, after some period of conventional treatment, you may need or want better control.

There are three common reasons to use intensive therapy:

1. You wish to approach normal blood glucose metabolism. The DCCT suggests that achieving nondiabetic blood glucose patterns may reduce the chance of complications, and intensive therapy can help you reach that goal. In addition, there's evidence that risks of birth defects are reduced when the mother's blood glucose is kept near nondiabetic levels. Thus, women who have diabetes and are pregnant or want to get pregnant often use intensive therapy.

2. Your diabetes is so unstable that, no matter how hard you try, you can't even come close to safe or adequate control. The reasons some people have so much difficulty while others manage easily are not always obvious.

3. You have an unpredictable lifestyle, such as changing work shifts or activity levels that fluctuate drastically from day to day or hour to hour. A standard program to anticipate insulin needs can't keep up with all the changes in your daily life, and a more adaptable and flexible program is needed.

Keep in mind, though, that intensive insulin therapy is a major undertaking, and using it to achieve normal blood glucose patterns is only recommended if you are highly motivated. It is *not* recommended for everyone! An intensified conventional plan might be a better option for some people.

## What additional resources do you need?

If you are embarking on an intensive diabetes treatment program, you need access to some very important health care resources. These include a physician (most likely an endocrinologist) who is experienced in treating people who are using intensive diabetes therapy, and an experienced diabetes nurse educator (most are actually certified diabetes educators, meaning they have significant experience and have passed a certification exam), who will help you understand many of the intricacies of making insulin adjustments, managing your condition on sick days, etc.

You will also want the services of a trained dietitian (many of whom are also certified diabetes educators) to help you develop an eating plan as part of your intensive therapy program. And you will, at different points in your journey to better diabetes control, be looking for the services of an exercise physiologist and even, perhaps, a psychosocial counselor for help in working through the challenges of intensive therapy.

## Summary

It's important that you carefully explore your reasons for undertaking this form of treatment. Discuss it in detail with your health care team before you decide. Any steps you can take to bring you closer to good physiologic control will be in the right direction. Success is closely linked with having the resources of a complete health care team at your disposal when needed. So be sure you don't start out on intensive therapy unless you have these important professionals available as part of your team.

# Chapter Two

# Designing Your Own Plan

- How do you set your goals?

- What do glucose patterns mean?

- What kind of schedule is right for you?

- Who's going to help and support you?

You can't start an intensive diabetes program the way you might start taking a new pill. The intensive plan requires a good bit of preparation. It's definitely not for impatient people!

- First, you must set treatment goals, usually based on the reasons for undertaking the intensive insulin therapy. You need to decide where you are heading before deciding how you will get there!
- Second, you must select which treatment regimen will be used. Your goals and the reasons you chose to intensify your therapy will often help you with this.
- Third, once you have made these decisions, you start a training program that will enable you to use your intensive program safely, comfortably, and successfully.

This last step can be the most challenging. It involves learning facts and procedures and also requires some "hands-on" training before you master the subtleties of your treatment program.

The reasons you undertake intensive diabetes therapy in the first place often dictate your goals of therapy.

## Normalizing glucose patterns

Perhaps you're choosing intensive therapy because you have high goals for your diabetes control. You want to achieve and maintain normal blood glucose metabolism. You may have targeted specific blood glucose levels or a glycohemoglobin value you want to achieve. Your goals are measured by specific numbers, with daily blood glucose values targeted to achieve a specific glycohemoglobin level.

Blood sugar ranges might be fasting levels of 70 to 110 mg/dl, prelunch and presupper values of 70 to 120, and levels one hour after meals under 180, two hours after meals under 150, and 3 A.M. levels over 65 mg/dl.

## Your glycohemoglobin goals

Most people with high goals define them in terms of a glycosylated hemoglobin value. This gives an average of blood glucose levels over the last two months. Your goal might be a value in or close to the nondiabetic range.

In the Joslin Diabetes Center clinical laboratory, the normal range for total glycosylated hemoglobin is 5.4 to 7.4 percent. Remember, the normal range in other laboratories may differ from that in the Joslin laboratory because these tests are performed in different ways in different places.

Realistically, glycohemoglobin values in the nondiabetic range might be difficult to achieve because of the increased risk for severe hypoglycemic (low blood sugar) episodes. In setting goals, you also should determine the frequency and severity of hypoglycemic reactions acceptable for you to maintain your safety. Most people achieve a successful balance between lowered glycohemoglobin and safety with a glycohemoglobin within about 20 percent of the upper limit of their laboratory's normal range. For the Joslin laboratory, this would be a glycohemoglobin of up to 8.9 percent.

Discuss your glycohemoglobin goal with your health care team and agree on a target. This level should be based on a realistic estimate of what you can achieve. You and your team can then plan how to lower your glycohemoglobin gradually and safely. Many people start intensive therapy because of unstable diabetes, with widely fluctuating glucose levels that conventional approaches haven't controlled. The goal is to get blood glucose levels closer to acceptable patterns, to eliminate severe low and high blood glucose levels and to help you feel better.

People with unpredictable lifestyles—those who seldom know when or what they'll eat or when or if they'll exercise—sometimes opt for the flexibility afforded by an intensive insulin program.

Here, the glycohemoglobin may not always tell the whole story. Since the glycohemoglobin represents an average of blood glucose levels, frequent high and low glucose values may average out to a "good" glycohemoglobin level but unacceptable patterns of control. In this case, undertaking intensive therapy to smooth out the patterns might actually *increase* the glycohemoglobin level. This is acceptable if you achieve your goal of compensating for daily variations and smoothing out the day-to-day patterns.

## Choosing an insulin dosing schedule

All intensive insulin plans allow you to adjust your insulin doses several times a day. Adjustments are based on blood glucose tests and other factors, such as how much you eat and how active you are. The objective is to reach a blood glucose level you and your physician have targeted. Various dosing programs are available. The major program types are outlined here.

### Intensified conventional therapy

• *Split-mix modifications.*—The simplest program for intensive insulin therapy is a variation of the conventional split-mix plan, by adjusting the regular insulin dose before breakfast and before supper (Figure 4).

Strictly speaking, this program falls short of true intensive insulin therapy because it only allows two, rather than three daily "decision points" to adjust the regular insulin dose. Many experts believe intensive therapy *must* use at least three daily decision points to provide even a minimal amount of flexibility. Nevertheless, this plan serves as an intermediate step between conventional and intensive therapy and may help some individuals who do not need or will not or cannot handle true intensive therapy.

For people with unstable diabetes, this program allows upward and downward dose adjustments for more aggressive glucose control. It is simpler to use than true intensive insulin programs. To intensify a split-mix program, you determine doses of regular insulin based on daily blood testing before breakfast and supper. You also occasionally need to test before lunch and before the bedtime snack at times.

Another way to use combinations of regular and intermediate (NPH or lente) insulins in an intensive insulin treatment program is the **three-injection variation of the split-mix:** regular plus an intermediate insulin in the morning, regular insulin at suppertime, and NPH or lente at bedtime.

On this regimen, you occasionally take regular insulin at bedtime along with the intermediate insulin if your glucose level at that time is high. Thus, technically, there are three times daily to give an adjustable regular insulin dose.

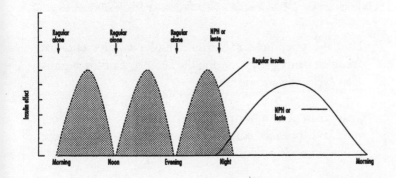

*Figure 4. The effect of a premeal regular insulin program with NPH or lente injection at bedtime. Regular insulin is injected before all three meals, with the intermediate-acting NPH or lente covering overnight.*

The later time of the second NPH or lente dose focuses more insulin effect during the latter part of your sleep cycle. At this time, usually about 4 or 5 A.M., changes in certain hormone levels (probably growth hormone) alter metabolism so you need more insulin. This rise in insulin requirements is called the "dawn phenomenon." If you have high fasting glucose levels, programs using bedtime intermediate insulin can be very effective.

## Multiple daily injections (MDI)

The multiple daily injections (MDI) plan is one of two approaches for intensive insulin therapy—the other being the use of an insulin pump. The MDI plan uses frequent insulin injections to mimic a normal pattern of insulin secretion throughout the day. Many combinations of insulins can be used, (details will be discussed in Chapter 6) but basic starting programs and their advantages are outlined below. Most people start intensive insulin therapy with an MDI program rather than a pump.

### What is the dawn phenomenon?

The dawn phenomenon is a rise in insulin requirements that occurs in many people during the latter part of the nightly sleep cycle, toward morning.

Changes in certain hormone levels (probably growth hormone and possibly cortisol) change metabolism so more insulin action is needed during this time.

People without diabetes can secrete this additional insulin as needed. But people using injected insulin may need to adjust their doses to compensate.

*Premeal regular and bedtime intermediate.*—This MDI program is popular with people who live unpredictable lifestyles. It uses regular insulin before each meal, with NPH or lente insulin as a fourth injection at bedtime (Figure 5). If you don't want to take four daily injections, you can take longer-acting ultralente insulin at supper time (three daily injections). With this program, the shorter and more predictable human form of ultralente is often the best choice.

Intermediate (or long-acting) insulins peak many hours after injection and may exhibit more variations in their peak times and duration than regular insulin. Therefore, dose adjustments of the longer-acting insulins may have a less precise effect than adjustments of regular insulin.

However, a program using premeal regular insulin and bedtime intermediate insulin permits three premeal dose decision points with nighttime coverage that is particularly effective for people with a prominent dawn phenomenon.

*Regular and ultralente.*—Another popular MDI program combines ultralente and regular insulin (Figure 5) to create insulin action patterns that more closely mimic normal patterns than other MDI schedules.

Ultralente is a long-acting insulin. Animal-source ultralente may last 24 to 36 hours or longer. In some people, some effect may persist for up to 96 hours. However, the newer human ultralente insulins tend to peak at about 12 hours and have exerted most of their effect within 24 hours.

When ultralente insulin is given once or twice a day, the action of successive doses overlaps, one almost fading into the next. These overlapping ultralente doses are effectively peakless and produce an almost constant basal insulin level. Additional injections of regular insulin before meals are based on blood glucose levels and adjusted for lifestyle variations.

There has been some concern that when regular insulin is mixed with ultralente, some of the regular is converted to a slower-acting form of insulin, reducing its rapid action. However, not mixing them would require five daily insulin injections rather than three. Injecting the insulin immediately after it is drawn up will minimize the loss of rapid action without requiring additional injections. (See Chapter 6 for more detail on this issue.)

When ultralente provides the basal insulin supply, the most common schedule is to give it with the prebreakfast and presupper regular insulin doses. Ultralente's basal action has a stabilizing effect on blood glucose control, so these programs may be useful for people with unstable diabetes or a variable lifestyle.

However, ultralente/regular programs are less effective than programs using nighttime intermediate insulin if you have a prominent dawn phenomenon. For this reason, some people may return to using bedtime NPH or lente if morning hyperglycemia persists.

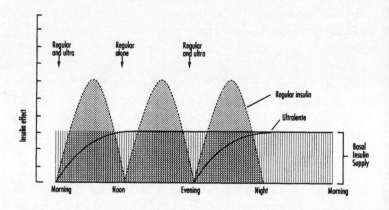

*Figure 5. The effect of an ultralente/regular insulin program for treating type I diabetes: ultralente is injected before breakfast and before supper, and regular insulin is injected before all three meals.*

Ultralente/regular programs may also be more difficult for people who regularly exercise strenuously. If you exercise and use ultralente you may have difficulty with hypoglycemia because ultralente's basal insulin supply may not dip low enough for the exercise or postexercise drops in glucose levels. This is known as the "lag effect." With a premeal regular and bedtime intermediate program, lower insulin levels can be designed for the proper times to prevent hypoglycemic reactions. Chapter 8 reviews these issues in more detail.

## Variations

Variations of these basic programs have been tried successfully to meet particular lifestyle or physiologic needs. An ultralente/regular program might be altered by giving NPH or lente instead of the twice daily utralente or as a substitute for either the morning or the evening ultralente to restore some of the peaking effect.

For example, changing presupper ultralente to bedtime NPH or lente provides a more prominent peak if you have fasting hyperglycemia due to the dawn phenomenon. Substituting intermediate for ultralente in the morning would provide the daytime basal plus a late afternoon or suppertime peak.

Conversely, substituting human ultralente, with a 12-hour peak, for intermediate provides prolonged action. Longer-acting insulin may also be given with the morning regular in a premeal regular and bedtime intermediate program to provide more of a basal effect. These various alternatives are discussed in Chapter 6 and outlined in Appendices 2 and 3.

## Pump programs

Continuous subcutaneous insulin infusion (CSII or the "pump") comes closest to mimicking normal insulin secretion patterns. The pumps now available don't measure blood glucose. You need to test your own blood, think about the result, decide on the proper insulin dose, and then program the pump.

Nevertheless, these pumps are reasonably effective at mimicking the pancreas's normal patterns of insulin secretion. They provide regular insulin through a catheter to a needle inserted just below the skin, usually on the abdominal wall or flank area. The user must replace the needle every two days.

The pump provides a slow, continuously absorbed flow of regular insulin that imitates the body's normal (basal) insulin pattern. Most pumps can be programmed to adjust the basal insulin flow at various times of the day or night. For example, more insulin can be infused during early morning as required by the dawn phenomenon.

Pumps also give short bursts of insulin, called boluses, before meals and snacks. As with the MDI programs, blood glucose measured at those times helps determine the quantity.

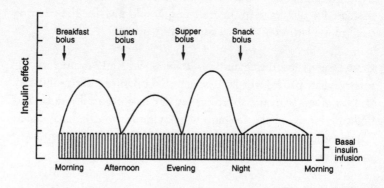

*Figure 6. Insulin effect seen when type I diabetes is treated with an insulin infusion pump. The constant regular insulin infusion provides the basal insulin supply. Boluses of regular insulin before meals and snacks cover insulin needs for incoming food.*

Pump treatment has all the advantages of MDI programs and delivers insulin in a manner that comes close to natural patterns. The insulin regimens are predictable, responsive, and flexible enough to accommodate lifestyle variations and the dawn phenomenon.

However, there are disadvantages, too. A pump sends a constant insulin flow into the body—day and night, in sickness or health, when active or sedentary, and when eating or starving! If the user skips meals or increases activity without changing the pump settings, hypoglycemia can occur.

Also, since there is no intermediate or long-acting insulin supplementing the regular insulin, any prolonged interruption of the pump insulin flow is likely to lead to a rapid rise in blood glucose and possibly ketoacidosis. Pumps require considerable attention and frequent self-blood glucose testing if they are to work effectively.

### Involving your management team

You must start and manage an intensive therapy program *only* with the assistance of a physician experienced in this type of treatment. Under *no* circumstances should anyone try to start his or her own intensive program based on knowledge gained from reading this manual or any other material. If fact, proper management of your intensive insulin program is best carried out by *more* than just a physician.

There are many advantages to the skilled diabetes management *team* that includes a physician, diabetes educator, dietitian, and others (such as an exercise physiologist and psychosocial professional) as needed. The DCCT study, in fact, demonstrated just how important regular interactions with the treatment team are. The nurse, dietitian, and other team members provide advice, guidance, expertise, and perhaps most important, support to the patients as they experience the ups and downs of intensive therapy.

While many physicians are capable of managing conventional insulin therapy, only those with special training should manage intensive therapy programs.

Improper or unsupervised intensive diabetes therapy may be less effective and is certainly more dangerous than even substandard conventional therapy. So if you choose intensive therapy, choose your health care team carefully.

Much of the "intensity" of intensive therapy comes from you. You need to become skilled at making routine management decisions about diabetes treatment, and you need to know how to handle any problems that might arise. Therefore, you must feel comfortable with your preparatory education before starting an intensive program.

Your education should begin with the basics, including a thorough understanding of diabetes—why it occurs, how we try to control it, and its potential complications. You need to be comfortable with all aspects of self-care—routine management, as well as the more complex and complicated problems.

It seems foolish for someone to start an intensive program, only to develop gangrene because he or she ignored a foot infection. Your knowledge of the topics covered in the rest of this book is essential for successful intensive therapy. Periodic updates and reviews keep your treatment up to date and prevent errors from creeping into your self-care routine.

For successful intensive therapy, you will need a thorough knowledge of self-monitoring of blood glucose (SMBG), including proper testing techniques and interpreting the results.

The use of meters is required. Their increased accuracy over visually read strips is crucial for success in intensive therapy. But meter use is only as accurate as the user's skill and care, so be sure you're properly taught how to use your meter and that you perform all tests correctly.

Discuss your choice of a meter with your health care team. To check your meter's accuracy, test your blood on your meter using the *same sample* sent to your doctor's lab and compare the simultaneous results.

Divide your meter results by 1.12 to convert this result on whole blood to the value you would get from blood plasma analyzed by most commercial laboratory methods. Also, remember that most self-testing meters, even after this calculation, may have a variation of up to 20 percent when compared with the lab test result.

Review your testing techniques periodically with your nurse educator. Bad habits can develop, even with the best of intentions, and a trained and certified diabetes nurse educator can spot and correct them.

## Testing schedule

For successful intensive insulin therapy, you should test your blood a minimum of four times daily—before each meal and at bedtime. These tests are essential to determine your next insulin dose and assess the previous one.

On occasions, to troubleshoot and assess program balance, testing at other times is important as well. Testing during the night—usually at about 2 or 3 A.M.—will help you differentiate among the various causes of fasting hyperglycemia. If you have fasting hyperglycemia and the 2 A.M. value is low, a nocturnal reaction with rebound hyperglycemia is possible.

On the other hand, a high value at 2 A.M. suggests insufficient overnight insulin coverage. A normal value during the night could mean the nighttime insulin isn't lasting long enough, or perhaps is peaking too early, with decreasing action later in the sleep cycle when more insulin is needed to counteract the dawn phenomenon.

You may also want to test one to two hours after meals to be sure that those blood glucose levels are not excessively high. Higher than expected glycohemoglobin levels with acceptable glucose values before meals and perhaps during the night are often due to high postprandial glucose levels. (See Chapter 3 for further discussion of how to use test information.)

## Record keeping

Keeping proper records is as important as actually doing the testing. You must maintain charts or booklets carefully, recording not only blood glucose levels, but also insulin doses, variations in activity and eating, stresses, and reactions. Often, writing down why you made certain insulin adjustments can build your management skills. These notes also help your health care team.

For monitoring records, list all test results for a given testing time in a column, so you can scan up and down for trends at that time over several days. You can also scan across the row to review glucose variations during that day. To the right of the day's blood glucose test results, list the insulin doses. (Doses can be placed along with the test results, but this is not as easy to scan.) In the far right column, leave space for comments. A sample of a monitoring record used at the Joslin Diabetes Center is included on page 238.

Avoid record logs that list all the glucose test results in a single column in the order you obtained them. This type of log makes it more difficult to identify trends for a particular time of day, for example prebreakfast glucose levels.

Also, "graph sheet" records may not be as useful as they seem. Besides not allowing scanning, graph sheets invite drawing lines between points. The lines imply, consciously or subconsciously, that the blood glucose level went from point A to point B directly. In reality, the level might have gone up or down or both, between these two points, so the implication of a direct line can be misleading.

Some of the newer meters have memories, which can be useful but can also be a crutch that promotes laziness by not forcing you to use written records. Keep in mind, flashing a readout of glucose numbers without dates, times, insulin doses, or comments is *useless!* Use your meter's memory only for short periods of time, if you are on the go and don't have your log book with you. Then, at the earliest opportunity, complete your handwritten log.

Even if you use a meter that outputs to a computer and allows data analysis, handwritten logs are still important. These logs are without equal in keeping you abreast of day-to-day variations and insulin needs. Computer analyses can be useful to analyze trends and patterns and pinpoint when blood glucose levels are highest or lowest, which helps with algorithm adjustments. Many people enjoy seeing the data they have diligently collected used to elucidate interesting patterns. Nevertheless, there is *no* substitute for careful, handwritten records!

## Ketones

It is also important that you know how to test for urine ketones, especially during an illness. Ketone testing helps you decide how much additional insulin is needed during "sick days." You should also know when to follow the rules for insulin supplementation, how to determine how much to give, and how to recognize when the need for increased monitoring and supplemental insulin has passed so you can return smoothly to your usual program.

An understanding of how to monitor during sick days is essential with both conventional and intensive therapies to avoid ketoacidosis and hospitalizations. Before you actually get sick, be sure to discuss sick-day monitoring and adjustment rules with your health care team. See Chapter 11 for details on how to use sick-day rules with intensive therapy.

## Back to basics

For someone undertaking intensive therapy, it may seem simplistic to spend time on basic skills of self-care and insulin use. Yet, these skills are of prime importance for all people with diabetes, and errors and misconceptions frequently creep into *everyone's* daily habits.

Carefully review proper insulin administration—it's performed incorrectly more often than you might imagine. If you use syringes, review proper measurement of insulin doses and administration of injections. Most physicians and diabetes educators recommend injecting 20 to 30 minutes before meals.

If you use a pump, be sure you understand catheter and needle use. Also, you should be intimately familiar with the workings of your pump, be able to troubleshoot minor problems, and know how to recognize major problems that require a temporary return to multiple injections. (See Chapter 7 for further discussion of pumps.)

### Your meal plan

You need to thoroughly understand the diabetic meal plan if you are to use any of the intensive therapies. Caloric intake is a major variable, and misunderstanding of dietary principles can doom any treatment program to failure.

While it is not within the scope of this manual to discuss the basics of a standard diabetic meal plan, the *use* of such a plan with intensive insulin therapy is discussed in Chapter 5. We strongly recommend that you consult a registered dietitian (RD) because improper or poorly followed meal plans are leading causes of failure of intensive diabetes therapy.

## The psyche and intensive therapy

Stress plays an important role in diabetes management, particularly if that stress distracts you from taking good care of yourself. This is another aspect of care you need to discuss with your diabetes team.

Also, explore how intensive diabetes therapy may add stress to your life. Discuss your expectations. Be sure they are realistic, and be prepared to cope with failure if you don't reach all of your goals. You may want to modify your goals if they are interfering with your quality of life.

Success is not guaranteed. We do not yet have a foolproof treatment for high blood glucose levels. It may be easy to accept this fact intellectually, but coping with it emotionally when this most intensive treatment fails to achieve your expected blood glucose goals can be frustrating and demoralizing.

Failing to achieve all of your initial goals is not *failure*. You are working at the edge of our technical and intellectual boundaries in the treatment of diabetes. You may not reach all your goals, but you have made a major step toward them. The more prepared you are for the inevitable setbacks, the better you will be able to cope and carry on. Some of these issues are discussed in greater detail in Chapter 10.

## Summary

Commit yourself to the philosophy of intensive therapy and the goals you and your health care team set. It takes a lot of time and effort to get the program running and to manage it with no guarantees that all of the desired goals will be achieved. However, intensive diabetes therapy affords greater flexibility along with improved diabetes control, plus the reasonable expectation that you will lower your chances of developing complications over the long haul. That's the payoff.

# Chapter Three

# Getting Started

## What's this section about?

- **What's an algorithm, anyway?**

- **How can this fit your lifestyle?**

- **What do we mean by blood glucose dynamics?**

- **How can you live with hypoglycemia?**

- **What is rebound hyperglycemia?**

## Understanding the algorithm

After your physician has worked with you to set your treatment goals and decide on a treatment program, the next step is selecting a starting insulin dosing plan.

Starting doses are usually estimates that take into consideration your previous insulin requirements, current level of control, or body weight. They may have no resemblance at all to where you end up, but they are a reasonable place to start.

Usually, your health care team will design an algorithm for insulin dose adjustments. Algorithms are charts that show you what specific dose of insulin should be given for a blood glucose level in a particular range. They are often designed by assigning a predetermined amount of insulin to the glucose range of about 100 to 150 mg/dl. Insulin doses are then moved up and down from that point.

For example, 1 or more units of regular insulin might be given for a glucose level of 150 to 200 mg/dl. Increments then are often 1-unit steps. Children may require only 1/2-unit steps, while some adults may require 2-unit steps or more. Occasionally, a glucose-level change doesn't require an insulin change.

You may need to be hospitalized to establish insulin doses and set up your personal algorithm, especially if you're going on an insulin pump. Not everyone needs to be hospitalized, however, and intensive outpatient programs are often recommended. Regardless of how you get started, the final treatment program is most effectively established over time as an outpatient.

## Intensive insulin therapy algorithm (sliding scale)

Insulin dose schedule for: _____

Date: _____ Clinic number: _____

**Regular insulin:**
*Your usual premeal insulin doses are:*

| Blood glucose | Breakfast | Lunch | Supper | Bedtime snack |
|---|---|---|---|---|
| 0–50 | ____ | ____ | ____ | ____ |
| 51–100 | ____ | ____ | ____ | ____ |
| 101–150 | ____ | ____ | ____ | ____ |
| 151–200 | ____ | ____ | ____ | ____ |
| 201–250 | ____ | ____ | ____ | ____ |
| 251–300 | ____ | ____ | ____ | ____ |
| Over 300 | ____ | ____ | ____ | ____ |

**Intermediate or long-acting insulin (NPH, lente, or ultralente):**

____    ____    ____    ____

### Smoothing out the patterns

When you're just beginning an intensive program, insulin doses should not result in extremely high or low glucose levels. But it's unlikely they will result in ideal glucose either. Usually, a number of adjustments will be needed. This "smoothing out" takes place as you live with your program. Keep in mind that perfect blood glucose levels are not essential at this stage.

It is often easier to smooth out your glucose patterns if you keep your blood glucose levels in the 150 to 250 mg/dl range, which isn't dangerous for short periods. By avoiding reactions, you also avoid the confusion that occurs when hyperglycemia (high blood glucose) follows a hypoglycemic reaction (low blood glucose). Then you need to figure out if the elevated glucose is related to rebound hyperglycemia, overfeeding the reaction, or insufficient insulin. If there are *no* reactions, hyperglycemia usually means there is too little insulin.

The first step in smoothing out your pattern is to adjust the insulin doses so glucose levels remain steady day and night. Then you can begin to carefully increase the amount of insulin so glucose levels fall to a more desirable range. Hypoglycemia is a common problem with intensive programs, so during this period, increases in the insulin dose must be made with forethought and caution.

### Adjusting the program to your lifestyle

Once you start your intensive program, get back to your usual lifestyle as soon as possible. Perhaps you have spent a few days in a hospital or you've taken time out from your usual routine to learn how to use intensive therapy. Such a break in the routine may have been important, but ultimately you must adjust your program to your lifestyle. In addition to insulin, you need to pay attention to your meal plan, activity, and daily schedule. Making intensive therapy part of your lifestyle can take weeks or even months.

But, unless you have unusual problems, there's no rush. In fact, taking your time incorporating intensive therapy into your daily life can be helpful; you gather more information to help you make decisions. Many people find this adjustment phase the most challenging part of the program.

During this period, you actually train yourself to make the daily adjustments of insulin, food, and activity to achieve your goals. You strive for independence so you won't have to depend on your health care team for decisions. You may well develop a "sixth sense" about how the different variables interrelate and how to balance them. At first, you depend on the algorithm, but ultimately you may go beyond this and make adjustments on your own, using the algorithm only as a guide.

So try to think beyond merely testing your blood and reading your algorithm. Consider the effects of what and when you've eaten, and how much activity you have had or will have.

For example, you might use one less unit of regular insulin because you exercised an hour earlier, or one more unit because your meal was larger than usual. You might use one more units because you'll be sitting in a meeting for the next four hours—or one less unit because the meeting may run late and delay your next meal!

You may wonder at this point, "How do I learn to consider all of these variables?" The answer is practice! No one starts intensive insulin therapy knowing how to make all of these adjustments. You must discover, through trial and error and working with your health care team, what works for you.

A five-mile jog might require a reduction of 4 units of insulin for one person, but a reduction of 2 units for another, to say nothing of the adjustments of food intake. The only way to learn what works for you is through *keeping good records of what you have done and how it affects your blood glucose levels.*

Focus first on blood sugars and insulin doses by meticulously regulating your eating and activity for the learning period. This eliminates these variables and allows you to pay close attention to just the insulin. If the sugars are high, you know it's not because of too much food or too little activity—you need more insulin.

Once you master the balance of insulin and blood glucose, you can add the other factors, such as food and exercise, into the equation. It will then be easier to appreciate the effects of these variables, and you can move beyond the algorithm into true intensive therapy.

## Understanding blood glucose dynamics

Keep in mind that blood glucose levels are constantly changing over the course of the day. A *single* blood glucose measurement tells you nothing about how and why glucose levels are changing.

It's like going to the seashore and taking a close-up photograph of the water level on a post. If you pointed to that photograph and said the water level is at that particular point on the post, your statement would be correct for just that one instant in time—but not for all time. You would be saying nothing about how fast or how much that water level had changed, how much it was likely to change, or what was causing it to change.

Think about how much more you would learn if you were to take a series of photographs and arrange them in the order they were taken. That would allow you to speculate more accurately about how the waves washed up and down against the post and how the tides rose and fell. You might also see evidence of a storm that temporarily raised the water level even more.

The more photographs, the more accurate your record. Of course, a video camera, constantly photographing the post, would give an even more precise picture of the dynamics of the water.

Think of your blood glucose tests as photographs, each freezing a single point in time. Like the photograph of the post in the water, each test represents one point on a dynamic sweep of glucose levels—moving up, down, or staying the same.

While we don't yet have anything similar to the video camera to follow constantly changing glucose levels, we can use multiple glucose tests to estimate those movements. With this information, plus knowledge about factors that affect glucose levels, we can estimate how far and how fast glucose levels are likely to change.

### Assessing direction and force of glucose movement

These two concepts—the direction the blood glucose level is moving and the force with which it moves—are crucial in understanding interactions and making appropriate adjustments.

At a given time, when the blood glucose level is at a specific point, various factors are exerting their effect on glucose in the blood. Depending on what those factors are, the glucose level may go up or down quickly or slowly.

### Sorting out the factors

To understand the direction and force of movement of glucose levels in your body, you need to think about all aspects of insulin's effect on glucose levels:

- Which insulin dose or doses are acting?
- Where is the insulin in its action curve? (Onset, peak, decline, etc.)
- How much insulin is working here?

With this information, you can estimate how the insulin is likely to affect the glucose levels. However, things can get more complicated because more than one factor may be affecting the blood glucose.

When several factors are at work, their effects may be additive. They can push the glucose level in the same direction or work opposite one another.

For example, both insulin and activity lower blood glucose levels. So when insulin is already moving the blood glucose down, activity will provide additional and stronger downward force. We already know this, of course. Exercising after an insulin injection can trigger a quick drop in blood glucose. This may be more pronounced when the insulin is peaking than when it's just beginning to act.

### Adding the concept of time

Time is another factor that must be included in the insulin–glucose equation. For example, let's say you inject regular insulin and then eat lunch 20 to 30 minutes later. As the food goes in, glucose moves slowly up. At this time, insulin is also moving slowly into the blood. So the forces are probably going to be roughly equal, and blood glucose won't change much.

An hour later, much of the food has been absorbed, and the glucose will be going up faster. More of the insulin is acting, too, but probably not as forcefully as the food. At this time, the glucose is probably higher than it was at mealtime. This is what we expect; the blood glucose level is higher one hour after a meal than it is before the meal. The larger the meal, the higher the blood glucose.

By three hours after the meal, much of the food has been absorbed and distributed to the cells of the body. At this point, regular insulin is approaching its peak action, so the downward force is greater than the upward force and blood glucose is dropping. Again, this is what we expect; the blood glucose will come back down about three hours after a meal.

## Understanding a hypoglycemic reaction

When blood glucose levels get too low, a hypoglycemic reaction occurs. The brain recognizes this crisis and sends out an SOS for "counter-regulatory hormones" (glucagon and epinephrine), which are secreted into the bloodstream. These hormones stimulate release of glycogen, a form of glucose stored in the liver and muscles. The glycogen is rapidly converted into glucose, resulting in a rise in blood glucose levels—the *rebound hyperglycemia* we see after a reaction.

A more severe reaction, causing more counterregulatory hormone secretion, might cause a more forceful rise in blood glucose. The upward rebound movement would be pushed by greater force, and the greater the force, the more rapid the uptrend and the higher it is likely to go.

The more upward force exerted, the more *downward* force it takes to counterbalance this, and the longer it might take for the rebound to subside. In fact, if no additional downward forces are added, the downtrend in the glucose levels may not occur until the upward force of the rebound has eventually dissipated. The higher glucose levels may persist for some time. Hence, while the actual upward *movement* of a rebound may last a relatively short time, it may take a while for the glucose level to come back down because the upward *force* has not yet been overcome.

Remember that this example is simplified. Usually, to complicate the picture, you also have other factors affecting glucose levels after a reaction, such as residual effects of previous activity and food consumed to treat the reaction. For these reasons, we usually advise people using conventional therapy not to "chase" rebound with more insulin. Additional insulin can cause too much downward force, leading to another reaction later.

## What is "rebounding" (the Somogyi effect)?

Rebounding, or the Somogyi effect (named after the physician who first described it), refers to high blood glucose levels (hyperglycemia) that follow a severe hypoglycemic reaction. Rebound usually occurs when the blood glucose falls to below normal levels. The body tries to compensate by releasing glucose stored by the liver as glycogen into the bloodstream. Sometimes the liver overdoes it and releases too much glycogen, producing elevated blood glucose levels.

Some people are more likely than others to experience rebounding. It is harmless—unless it is misunderstood, in which case someone may give you more insulin, when in fact you need less.

There is no usual pattern to rebounds but they may last 12 to 24 hours after a severe hypoglycemic reaction. The resulting upward swing of blood glucose levels can last even longer. This condition usually corrects itself if left alone. You should not use extra insulin to lower the blood glucose unless the high levels continue for several days. And be sure you eat normal amounts of food during rebounds.

The danger comes from giving still more insulin or eating too little. That can make the blood glucose level drop and start the same cycle over again. If the symptoms of hypoglycemia aren't obvious, check your blood glucose often to see if you can discover a pattern.

## Applying these concepts to real life

Understanding the theory we've outlined here may be relatively easy. But to master the concepts as they apply to you, you must carefully study the results of your frequent monitoring.

As you look at each test, try to decide what factors have provided the downward forces: insulin, exercise, reduced eating? What caused the upward forces: rebound, illness, overeating, underactivity?

Of course, many factors affect blood glucose levels, and some are difficult to recognize. It is also difficult to estimate the force each exerts. Making these estimates takes experience, patience, and time.

By repeatedly seeing the effects on glucose levels of given amounts of insulin, food, and activity, you can learn how these factors affect *you* and then adjust them accordingly. Review your test results with the diabetes team to help you learn to make proper interpretations. When patterns are not clear, even an experienced observer may need many days of data to discover general trends. Days that "just don't make sense" can be disregarded.

Sometimes it helps to study certain variables more precisely by reducing the effect of other factors on blood glucose levels. Hypoglycemia and rebound or feeding hyperglycemia often cause confusion. The patterns might be easier to spot if you let your blood glucose run a little high (perhaps 150 to 250 mg/dl before meals) or carefully control activity and food consumption for a while.

Although the dose changes set up for you on your personal algorithm will compensate for glucose levels that aren't within your target range, never assume the algorithm will *automatically* fix aberrations or compensate for very unusual eating or activity. Always try to determine what combination of factors caused the glucose level to change.

## The importance of record keeping

As we have said, proper record keeping is crucial. Your records must include not only blood glucose levels and insulin doses, but also notes about deviations from normal eating and activity patterns.

It's often helpful to quantitate variations from a "normal" day. Estimate how much activity and food is normal, then indicate variations by noting "-2" for much less, "-1" for a little less, "+1" for a little more, and "+2" for a lot more.

Write these notations in the "comments" section of your record book, along with the time the variation occurred and any other unusual circumstances. Then you can scan the record days later and have a simple way to identify variations and relate them to insulin or glucose changes. (See pages 237 to 239 at the back of the book for a sample record.)

## Summary

Hit-and-miss record keeping won't help you or your team understand why you were high one day or low two days later. The intensive approach requires a commitment to careful detective work. No clue should be overlooked.

Once your intensive plan becomes a natural part of your life, you'll be able to state *why* you were high or low on a given day. Your medical team can give you information and tools. But only you can make intensive therapy work!

# Living with an Intensive Plan

There is no clear line between the end of the start-up phase and the beginning of living the rest of your life with intensive diabetes therapy. As you gain experience, you gradually set your sights beyond immediate accomplishments and toward your ultimate treatment goal of blending your diabetes care into your daily routine.

Even after the initial start-up period, intensive diabetes programs may still require adjustments. Seasonal lifestyle variations, changes in job or routine, and the effects of aging all can affect the treatment program.

## Modifying your program

Adjustments of intensive diabetes algorithms are more complex than the standard adjustments for conventional therapy. Insulin algorithms may be designed to move a given blood glucose level, regardless of what it is, toward a specifically targeted range.

Adjustments can compensate for variations caused by such things as depth of injection, food absorption, and air temperature, often not identifiable and usually beyond our control. Still, these programs are designed to *anticipate* a fairly *routine* eating and activity pattern. If you ignore changes in eating and activity and assume the algorithm will automatically compensate for even excessive variability, the program may not work well.

The key phrase, however, is *beyond our control*. Most diabetes management plans assume a "usual" diet and activity level—the factors that we *do* control. The purpose of intensive therapy is *not* to allow total disregard of, or a haphazard approach to, eating and activity. So, before making any insulin dose changes, be sure you have eliminated exercise or eating as causes of fluctuating blood glucose.

Once you rule out eating and exercise as the cause of high or low blood glucose levels, you can modify your insulin algorithm using one of two approaches. The first is to consider this entire range of doses as a *single* dose, even though each is actually designed to bring a different range of glucose values toward a targeted level. The other approach is to view the algorithm as a series of *different* doses, one for *each* glucose level, and each to be treated differently.

To decide which approach to take, determine why the target blood glucose levels are not being reached.

• First, rule out diet or exercise variations.

• Next, examine your test results and determine whether the failure occurs at *all* glucose levels or just at *some* levels. Is there a *consistent* defect in the effect of insulin doses in the algorithm, regardless of the starting level?

Using the algorithmic scale, if you fail consistently to reach the target glucose level and the error is *always* (or almost always) in the same direction (always too high or always too low), then the whole scale is off-target consistently. Therefore, think of the whole scale as *one* dose and increase or decrease the quantities of *all* insulin doses for each blood glucose level up and down the scale.

However, with sliding scales, part of the scale may work well while another part does not. For example, assume that for blood glucose levels above 180 mg/dl, the prescribed doses work well at bringing the blood glucose levels down to 80 to 120 mg/dl by the next test period. However, when the starting glucose is under 180, you have difficulty with hypoglycemic reactions a few hours later. The adjustment, therefore, must be in the insulin doses on the *lower end of this scale only*. Doses for starting values above 180 mg/dl remain unchanged.

To adjust individual parts of the scale, think of the sliding scale as a group of *many* doses rather than as a *single* dose. Each dose is assigned to a specific range of starting blood glucose levels. Obviously, you must accumulate information for several days so you have enough to analyze individual insulin doses at various glucose level ranges.

In trying to do this type of analysis, hypoglycemic reactions and rebound or overfeeding hyperglycemia can be very confusing. They make the responses to a given insulin dose in a particular blood glucose range seem inconsistent.

If you suspect undetected hypoglycemic reactions, you may want to reduce your overall dose, as suggested earlier. In this case, temporarily reduce the basal—the pump basal or the ultralente dose, for example—to allow sugars to rise to that 150 to 250 mg/dl range that allows a clearer look at the patterns. Doing so will eliminate reactions and allow better dose adjustment.

By eliminating the inconsistency, the answer to the question, "Is that sugar high because not enough insulin was given or because of rebound?" will always be "Not enough insulin!" Later on, glucose levels can be returned to target ranges by going back to the higher basal or ultralente doses.

In general, the first objective is to smooth out the patterns. Once the patterns are smooth, the next objective is to bring the overall glucose levels down to the acceptable levels by increasing the appropriate individual insulin doses.

### Routinely compensating for the variables

The above approach is most useful in fine tuning an intensive insulin program or adapting one to a changed lifestyle. However, once your program is established and working smoothly, you may still need to adjust it on a given day to accommodate for major changes in eating or activity. While the algorithm should routinely compensate for *minor* changes, significant alterations require further adjustment.

For example, you can anticipate planned activity variations, such as the Tuesday evening basketball game or the Thursday morning aerobics class, by reducing the algorithmic dose of regular insulin taken just before that activity. You determine the degree of variation by trial and error, with proper record keeping so you can learn from your experience. To start with, however, you may try reducing each value on the scale by one unit.

Picture the variables and resulting adjustments schematically. Remember, your goal is to maintain smooth blood glucose levels. The forces affecting your blood glucose levels after a normal breakfast are shown in Figure 7-A, on the next page. There would be an upward force from the food you have eaten and a downward force from the insulin.

Figure 7-B shows the same insulin and breakfast, but adds the effect of a morning exercise class. With this activity, the net effect is now a downward movement of the blood glucose level, with the chance of a reaction.

You have three options for reducing the chances of a drop in the blood glucose level, and these options are the same whether you are using intensive, intensified conventional, or conventional therapy. First, eat extra food to compensates for the exercise (Figure 7-C). Second, take less insulin (see Figure 7-D). Or, third, you can do both.

This example illustrates that an algorithm is primarily designed to compensate for some of the intangible factors that affect blood glucose levels. Exercise, however, adds an *anticipatory* part of diabetes control program.

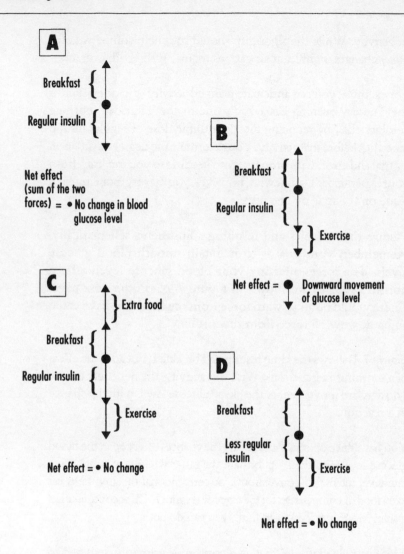

*Figure 7.* *(A) The upward force on your blood glucose level after a normal breakfast. If your insulin dose is calculated properly, the upward force from the food should be equal to the downward force from the insulin, and the glucose level should not rise significantly. (B) Forces affecting the same insulin and breakfast, but adding a morning exercise class, which increases the downward force, leading to a drop in the glucose level. (C) How extra food will compensate for the exercise to maintain a steady glucose level. (D) How less insulin will reduce the downward force and maintain a steady glucose level.*

By anticipating the effect of something that will alter your blood glucose, you can compensate for it, rather than ignoring it and hoping that the algorithm will fix the problem at the next decision point.

Of course, it isn't always so simple! Many people on a *regular* exercise program notice only minimal changes in blood glucose levels when activity is stopped for a day or two. Adjustments based on the algorithm are often all that is needed.

After exercise, the body needs to rebuild glycogen supplies (a stored form of glucose), which can lead to hypoglycemia a number of hours later in some people. This is called the "lag effect." If your exercise, watch for this. You may need more food after exercise, or you may need to reduce your insulin dose.

Pump users who exercise intensely often take their pumps off when the exercise starts, keep them off during the exercise, and sometimes don't put them on for a while after exercise. All these adjustments become much easier with time—after you've learned how your treatment program works for you. (Details on exercise and intensive insulin therapy can be found in Chapter 8.)

## Dealing with specific problems

While each person using intensive insulin therapy requires individual adjustments and treatment modifications, general guidelines are useful. General approaches for treating common glucose control problems are discussed below. In addition, specific guidelines can be found in Appendices 7, 8, and 9.

## Hyperglycemia

Blood glucose levels that are too high (hyperglycemia) are treated by increasing the insulin dose providing primary coverage for that time period. When you use premeal *regular* insulin, the doses are designed to control blood glucose levels from the time of that meal through the period just after the meal (the postprandial period), and up to just before the next meal (or bedtime, in the case of the presupper dose).

If you are using conventional therapy and your glucose levels are consistently too high at a certain time of the day, an increase of the premeal dose that covers that time is the obvious solution. If elevated fasting blood glucose is the problem, you can treat it by increasing the basal insulin supply (pump basal, ultralente, or bedtime intermediate insulin doses).

Unfortunately, decisions may be more complicated with intensive insulin therapy because there are more choices of insulin doses to alter. One insulin's action may overlap the action of the next. You must also consider food and activity. Appendix 6 details the approach to hyperglycemia for the standard intensive insulin treatment programs.

Here's an example of how to approach hyperglycemia. Consider a high postlunch glucose level that has come down to the target level by dinnertime. A simple prelunch dose increase might lower the postmeal glucose level but could lead to hypoglycemia before supper. Another option would be to change the composition of the lunch meal by reducing carbohydrate.

Also, look at the timing of the insulin dose. It is ideally given 20 to 30 minutes before eating. If blood glucose is too high after you eat, perhaps allowing more time between the insulin dose and the meal will allow more of the insulin to be available for the incoming carbohydrate.

Another alternative is to increase the insulin dose and add a supplemental snack at the peak insulin time to prevent hypoglycemia. Perhaps you can adjust the timing of the meal as well.

Finally, remember that insulins do not act within strict times. They are affected by any other insulin that has been injected.

Previous insulins may still be exerting their waning effects on blood glucose levels when the next insulin dose comes into play. For example, longer-acting insulins such as NPH or lente injected with regular may begin acting about the same time the regular is peaking, pushing blood glucose levels down further than they might go without this overlap. Adjustment of either of these might be helpful.

Knowing all of these possible approaches to the problem, you must then decide which will work best. First, identify which of the possible causes is actually responsible.

## The dawn phenomenon and rebound

Fasting hyperglycemia is usually caused by insufficient insulin duration overnight (the dawn phenomenon), or rebound of hyperglycemia after marked hypoglycemia (the Somogyi phenomenon.) Hyperglycemia at other times of the day may be caused by not enough insulin or insulin that doesn't last long enough, diet or exercise variations, or hypoglycemia and rebounds. Appendix 7 lists glucose test patterns that can help you determine the cause of the problem.

Next, once you know the reason for the hyperglycemia, you can decide which adjustment will work best. If your diet is incorrect, adjust it. If not enough insulin is available, increase it, adding a snack later in the afternoon if necessary.

When making these adjustments, use systematic trial and error, with proper record keeping so you know what you have done and how it has worked. Be as consistent as possible in considering all the variables that affect diabetes control.

### Hypoglycemia

Low blood glucose (hypoglycemia) is a common problem because attempts to maintain normal blood glucose can lead to taking more insulin than you actually need. Nighttime hypoglycemia followed by hyperglycemic rebound can cause fasting hyperglycemia. When low blood glucose is a problem, make every attempt to identify the timing of the hypoglycemia and record this information in your record book.

Keep in mind that some symptoms could be signs of something other than hypoglycemia. Many of the so-called hypoglycemic symptoms, such as sweats and shakes, are caused by adrenalin secretion triggered by falling blood glucose and are not a direct effect of the low glucose level itself. Fear, anxiety, or even a rapidly dropping (but not abnormally low) blood glucose level can also trigger adrenalin secretion and can produce symptoms without true hypoglycemia. Therefore, try to document true hypoglycemia by testing your blood.

Also, as control improves and is close to normal more often, some people find that their symptoms of hypoglycemia become more subtle. In some cases, they may not even know they are having a hypoglycemic reaction until they become disoriented or unconscious. For these reasons, people on intensive insulin therapy need to learn how and when to anticipate these lows. Also, they need to teach their loved ones how and when to administer glucagon, and teach their friends and family how to recognize these signs of hypoglycemia and what to do in case of a severe low.

When you know you have actually had a hypoglycemic reaction, first treat the reaction immediately. Treatment options are discussed in Appendix 8, with specific foods listed in Appendix 9. In general, as long as you are conscious, eating some rapidly absorbable carbohydrate is the first step.

People taking insulin, especially those using an intensive approach, should always have an easily consumed carbohydrate with them, such as tablets, sugar, or Lifesavers® (see Appendix 9 for a more complete list). If you aren't planning a meal or snack within an hour after the hypoglycemic reaction, eat a slowly absorbed carbohydrate as well, such as bread or crackers.

On the rare occasions when you can't think clearly or are unconscious, orally ingestible carbohydrate should be avoided because it may be inhaled into the lungs. Family members or friends can give glucagon if they have been trained to do so. If they can't do this, or if the glucagon doesn't work, you need to be taken to an emergency facility immediately for intravenous glucose.

## Explained and unexplained reactions

After the hypoglycemia is corrected, carefully analyze events leading up to it to determine why it happened. There are two types of hypoglycemic reactions: "explained" and "unexplained."

*Explained hypoglycemic reactions* occur for identifiable reasons—you missed a meal, you had an unexpected increase in activity, or you used too much insulin. Document these reactions. Note whether the problem was an error in technique (inadvertently giving too much insulin) or an error in judgement (not reducing insulin to compensate for activity or less food).

If you can't find the cause of the hypoglycemia, it is an *unexplained reaction*, which *may* mean your basic insulin dose (regular, basal, or both) is too high. However, the reaction also may result from a number of intangible factors on that given day, while on other days the same dose is just fine.

For example, slightly more activity, plus slightly more rapid insulin absorption, slightly slower food absorption, and a slightly lower glucose level may, when combined, have too great a downward force on the glucose level.

If the hypoglycemic reaction was severe, reduce the insulin dose that was most probably at fault for the next day. If the reaction was mild and you have had no serious problems in the past with the same dose, do not change it. (*Note:* This may differ from instructions given with conventional insulin therapy, and it may be different for people using intensive diabetes therapy for the primary purpose of avoiding severe reactions.)

Over the next few days, monitor your blood glucose carefully to reconfirm that the hypoglycemic reaction was indeed just a one-time aberration. If reactions occur again at the same time or if patterns show a repeated drop in glucose levels at that time, the dose should be reduced.

If you aren't sure what's happening, it never hurts to reduce the insulin dose by a unit or two and carefully watch the effect. Remember, however, that people who have ambitious goals for blood glucose levels will have occasional hypoglycemic reactions, no matter how careful they are. These reactions are risks that are hopefully offset by the benefits. So, don't compromise your attempts at intensive control for the sake of eliminating mild, manageable hypoglycemic reactions.

What are acceptable frequency and severity of reactions? Discuss this with your health care team. Loss of consciousness or reactions in which you're unable to function appropriately must be avoided, no matter what your goals are.

How do you determine the specific insulin or the dose that caused the hypoglycemic reaction? Initially, assume that the hypoglycemia results from too much insulin peaking closest to the time of the reaction. For example, a reaction before lunch would have been caused by too much prebreakfast regular insulin. (See Chapter 7 for further discussion.)

However, determining the actual insulin dose at fault may not always be this easy. If adjustment of the obvious dose doesn't correct the problem, leads to other problems, or fails to stop the reactions, you need to consider other possibilities. Remember, insulin actions can overlap.

For example, with a simple split-mix pattern (using regular plus NPH or lente before breakfast), you can assume that hypoglycemia at 11:30 A.M. has been caused by the morning regular insulin. But say this mixture was injected at 6:30 A.M. The blood glucose levels at 11:30 A.M., five hours after injection, would reflect both the post-peak regular insulin's waning action and the intermediate insulin's increasing effect.

Figure 8 and 9 illustrates this point. Figure 8 shows the overlap between morning regular and NPH or lente during the prelunch period. Figure 9 shows the effect of downward forces from the regular plus the intermediate insulins. The overall effect is greater than the effect of one of these insulins alone. This phenomenon is often very clear for people using the newer human insulins, which tend to act more reliably at their expected times.

Hypoglycemia before lunchtime can result from either insulin or both, and adjustment of either insulin might correct the problem. Decide which insulin to adjust based on blood glucose levels at the peak times of each insulin or the ratio of the regular to the intermediate insulin.

For example, if your blood glucose level at the peak of the regular insulin was relatively low, but the level was on the high side when the NPH or lente was peaking, you might reduce the regular insulin. On the other hand, if the dose of regular is already small in

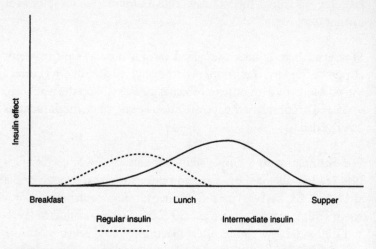

*Figure 8.* The insulin effect seen when a mixed morning dose of regular plus intermediate insulin is taken.

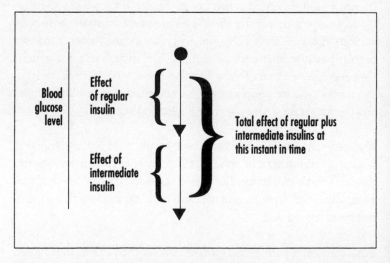

*Figure 9.* The additive effect of the morning regular and intermediate insulins just before lunch. The total downward force on the glucose level is made up of the sum of the downward force from the waning regular insulin action curve plus the downward effect of the beginning of the intermediate insulin action curve.

relation to the NPH, the effect of the regular insulin may still be less important than that of the NPH or lente.

If you reduce the regular insulin, you might be left with such a small morning dose of regular insulin that meaningful future adjustments could be difficult. A change of even one unit would be a large percentage of the total dose of regular insulin. Therefore, in this instance, reducing the NPH or lente is preferable.

If you undertake a true intensive insulin program, it's important that you understand the adjustment concepts outlined above. However, in order to appreciate them, you need to experience some of the problems and find solutions for yourself. Your physician or diabetes educator can use your blood test results to help you decide on how to make adjustments

## Weight gain

The goal of intensive therapy is to improve diabetes control. This means calories previously lost as sugar in the urine become available to use as energy, or to be stored as fat!

If you gain weight after starting intensive therapy and the weight isn't from fluid retention that can accompany sudden improvements of diabetes control, you may need to change your diet and lower the total calorie level. With fewer calories, you may need less insulin. Work with your dietitian to decrease the likelihood of weight gain.

If your intensive insulin program is improperly designed or calls for too much insulin, you might be eating "to feed your insulin." The insulin may lower your glucose too much, creating a need to eat to keep blood levels in the target range. In this case, a little less insulin might help reduce the amount of food you eat. Work with your nurse educator and your exercise physiologist to identify ways of addressing this.

## Summary

Once your intensive diabetes program has started, it is important to mold your treatment to your body's metabolic needs. The next step is to balance your metabolic needs with some degree of lifestyle flexibility. Understanding how the various insulin work, alone and as part of your daily treatment plan, will help you "fine tune" your self-management skills.

# Chapter Five

# Planning Your Meals

- Why think about food as fuel?

- What's so important about timing?

- Is this snack necessary?

- What about stuff like fiber, weight control, carbohydrate counting, sick days, alcohol, and the glycemic index?

Food is the fuel our bodies need for energy to run the organs that keep us alive and the muscles that keep us going. Insulin-dependent diabetes prevents the cells of the body from getting the fuel they need (energy in the form of glucose) because of a lack of insulin. So the challenge facing people with diabetes is to replace that missing insulin—the right amount at just the right time for just the right amount of incoming glucose to provide energy for a given activity and metabolic needs. This is truly a balancing act!

We have discussed how conventional insulin therapy is based upon predictable activity, food (fuel) intake, and metabolic needs from one day to the next, while intensive insulin therapy allows for variability of these factors. Thus, with intensive insulin therapy, rigid meal plan adherence to choice of foods and the timing of meals may be relaxed somewhat. However, it is important to remember the principles!

## Food as the body's fuel

To understand how food affects the blood glucose control you are striving for, it helps to review how food provides for our nutritional needs and plays a role in our metabolism.

The U.S. Dietary Goals are nutritional guidelines that apply to all individuals, whether or not they have diabetes. They state that we should all:

1. Eat a variety of foods every day.
2. Maintain desirable weight.
3. Choose a diet low in fat, saturated fat, and cholesterol.
4. Choose a diet with plenty of vegetables, fruits, and grain products.
5. Use sugar in moderation.
6. Use salt and sodium only in moderation.
7. If you drink alcoholic beverages, do so in moderation.

## Digestion and gastric emptying

Digestion, the breakdown of foods in the gastrointestinal tract, occurs at different rates for different foods. Digestion actually begins in your mouth, where your teeth break up larger food particles and saliva begins the breakdown of carbohydrates into individual sugar molecules. The digestive activity of the saliva continues until it is inhibited by the acid in the stomach.

Stomach acid and enzymes continue the digestion of food. Certain enzymes break down certain types of food. For example, pepsin digests proteins into their basic components, amino acids. Very little absorption of food into the blood stream occurs in the stomach. However, substances that we all know can "get into your bloodstream fast," such as alcohol and aspirin, do so because they *are* absorbed in the stomach. Thus, if you drink alcohol, it is better to do so with food, which slows down absorption.

Digested food passes next into the duodenum, the first portion of the small intestine. This is called "gastric emptying." The rate of gastric emptying can be affected by the composition of the stomach contents. For example, when the stomach contains fat, acid, very concentrated (hypertonic) solutions, or is distended, emptying is slowed or delayed.

Fat is the most potent inhibitor of gastric emptying, and a meal with significant amounts of fat will delay gastric emptying. Some of the meal will still be in the stomach six hours later! By contrast, a meal consisting primarily of protein and carbohydrate may empty in three hours. Fat and protein can stimulate the secretion of two hormone substances called secretin and cholecystokinin, which slow gastric emptying. Dietary fiber may also slow gastric emptying.

Gastric emptying rates are important to people with diabetes because the slower the gastric emptying, the slower the nutrients are absorbed, and the slower the rise in blood glucose levels.

For people with diabetes, slowly rising blood glucose levels are preferable, of course; they are more easily coordinated with injected insulin. That is why we emphasize meals with a combination of protein, carbohydrate, and fat. It is also why we may manipulate your diet—to change absorption rates in an effort to prevent troublesome variations in glucose levels after you eat.

## Carbohydrate

Carbohydrate is made up of many sugar molecules, and is the primary energy source for our bodies, providing 4 calories per gram of sugar. It is found in milk, vegetables, fruits, and other starchy foods. Dietary carbohydrates are broken down into their basic building blocks, sugars. The breakdown and absorption is rapid, and most dietary carbohydrate is absorbed by the time it reaches the end of the second portion of the small intestine, the jejunum.

You may have been taught in the past by your health care team that there are different types of carbohydrates (simple and complex) and that these are absorbed at different rates. Evolving recommendations from the American Diabetes Association (ADA) suggest that the differences between these two groups are far less significant than previously thought, however. Equal amounts of carbohydrates, regardless of their source, have the same effect on blood sugars, the ADA states in new recommendations released in the spring of 1994.

As glucose from dietary carbohydrate flows into the blood stream, it usually provides for the immediate energy needs. Much of the excess glucose energy not immediately needed can be stored as glycogen, a substance similar to a carbohydrate. Glycogen is stored in the liver and muscle and can be mobilized quite rapidly when energy from glucose is needed. Further excesses of glucose can be converted into fats and stored for later needs.

## Protein

Dietary protein is first broken down into peptide fragments, which are split apart further into amino acids, the basic constituent of proteins. These amino acids are absorbed into the bloodstream from the small intestine.

About 58 percent of the ingested protein will be converted into sugar, so protein indirectly can also be a source of energy. Like carbohydrate, protein provides an energy supply of 4 calories per gram. The rest of the amino acids go to provide for the body's protein needs.

## Fat

Most of the fat consumed is digested and absorbed into the bloodstream from the small intestine. Fat is in the diet as triglycerides, phospholipids, and cholesterol. When digested, fat is broken down into its constituents: free fatty acids and monoglycerides. Once absorbed, fatty acids are resynthesized into triglycerides.

Triglycerides plus small amounts of phospholipid, cholesterol, free fatty acids, and protein, form small droplets called chylomicrons, which flow through the blood. After a fatty meal, therefore, blood plasma may appear milky because of the presence of these chylomicrons. Fat is a very dense storage form of energy, and, when metabolized, provides 9 calories per gram.

As a meal is absorbed, most of the energy supplied comes from glucose. The amino acids and fat are used to replace body proteins and structural fats that have been degraded by the body's natural processes.

However, amino acids, fats, and a large portion of the carbohydrates *not* used for energy are converted to tissue fat—the body's way of storing this energy surplus for later use (we hope!). In the postabsorptive state—after all the eaten food is absorbed and no stream of glucose flows in from the gastrointestinal tract—the body can turn to stored energy from glycogen or fat to provide for its needs.

## The meal plan

As you can see, digestion is accomplished through a series of processes regulated by the body. Your participation in the process will be the selection and consumption of a healthy diet. The first step in developing a meal plan is an interview with a qualified dietitian. Professional assistance is the best way for you to have a plan designed for *you,* based on your individual needs and food preferences.

The process begins with an evaluation of how well your current eating patterns meet your nutritional and medical needs. The dietitian will assess weight gain or loss, personal food preferences, amounts of time available for food preparation, and timing and size of usual meals. This information about your eating style allows the development of a nutrition profile containing information for the physician and a recommended meal plan for you.

Calorie levels for the meal plan will be based on previous eating habits, with a decrease in calories if you need to lose weight. The dietitian and physician will also use several other guidelines to estimate calorie needs. For example, ideal body weight can be estimated by the following calculations:

| | |
|---|---|
| *Males:* | 106 pounds for the first 5 feet of height |
| | 6 pounds for each additional inch over 5 feet |
| *Females:* | 100 pounds for the first 5 feet of height |
| | 5 pounds for each additional inch over 5 feet |

This calculation may be increased or decreased by a factor of 10 percent, based on larger or smaller frame sizes. Dietitians can then adjust calorie intake, based on your actual weight compared with ideal weight, to help you reach your weight goals.

## Composition of meals

In the past, when physicians realized that diabetes prevents proper metabolizing of carbohydrates, they logically recommended a diet low in carbohydrate—and thus high in fat.

More recently, your dietitian may have recommended to you a ratio of carbohydrate-to-protein-to-fat of something like 50 percent to 20 percent to 30 percent.

New guidelines being released by the American Diabetes Association recommend that the development of a meal plan and the distribution of calories and nutrients be more individualized than this. They should be based on the individual's usual eating style, as well as his or her blood glucose and lipid (blood fat) control. Recommendations that dictate a distribution of nutrients as a percent of total calories do not allow for individual variation and needs.

The 1994 ADA nutrition recommendations state that protein should contribute 10 to 20 percent of total calories and saturated fat should be less than 10 percent of total calories. The level of carbohydrate and unsaturated fats should be determined based on individual considerations.

If, for example, you have an elevated triglyceride level, you may find a diet high in carbohydrate worsens your triglycerides as well as your blood sugar control. On the other hand, if you have elevated LDL cholesterol levels, or if your priority is to lose weight, you may respond best to a low-fat meal plan.

Adjustments in sodium in your meal plan also is important. While sodium does not affect blood sugar levels, some people are affected by high salt levels—which shows up as fluid retention or high blood pressure. For this reason, sodium levels no higher than 3 grams per day are recommended.

Fiber continues to be an important part of your diet. The high-fiber fruits and vegetables in a typical diabetes meal plan help you feel full and satisfied—something that often doesn't happen with highly processed foods. So your dietitian will encourage you to eat 20 to 35 grams of fiber daily.

Developing a comfortable, healthy eating pattern is a process that may take a while. Changes don't have to be made all at once; you can make adjustments over time. Dietitians provide plans for gradually changing eating patterns by working with recipes and prescribing stepwise changes. The key to success lies in working with your diabetes care team.

### Timing

Consistency of meal and snack times, while often less rigid with intensive diabetes therapy, is still important. A theoretical advantage of intensive insulin therapies, especially pump therapy, is the flexibility in the timing of meals.

However, the consequences of mealtime variations differ among the various intensive diabetes programs and the levels of glucose sought. Programs with significant percentages of the daily insulin supply in the basal component (such as pump therapy or ultralente) tend to be more forgiving of timing variations.

It is important that you coordinate the action of your insulin with your daily food consumption. As you are becoming familiar with the use and adjustment of your insulin algorithm, you should be as consistent as possible with the timing and selection of meals and snacks.

This is especially true when using intermediate insulins. They have pronounced peaks, and with a duration of action that is fairly long, it can be difficult to estimate at injection time exactly how much insulin will be needed later in the day when the insulin is peaking.

If the timing of a meal is significantly delayed, then the premeal dose of regular insulin may also be delayed. However, you should eat some of the carbohydrate portion of the meal—some starch or fruit—before the meal.

If your glucose levels are in the normal range, they may drop too low by meal time. If the delay is to extend to a couple of hours, then you may wish to switch the meal with the snack that was to have been eaten several hours after that meal. Eat the snack at meal time and the meal at the time the snack was to have been eaten. The insulin dose may also need to be adjusted.

You should discuss with your health care team in advance how to handle this type of situation.

Meals and snacks should ideally be spaced at least two to three hours apart so digestion can occur. Blood sugar can then rise and fall again before more food is eaten. If snacks are too close to a meal, the blood sugar will still be high when the meal is eaten and the blood sugar after the meal will probably be higher than desired—unless other adjustments are made.

### Snacks

Between-meal and evening snacks are important to help counter the effect of insulin acting over long stretches of time or with increases in activity.

Snacks may be incorporated into the meal plan at specific times, usually midmorning, afternoon, and evening, depending on the interval between meals and the action times of your prescribed insulin program. Bedtime snacks that contain protein and carbohydrate prevent hypoglycemia during the night. Midmorning and afternoon snacks may help prevent drops in the glucose level if there are long intervals between meals.

For example, if several hours pass between an afternoon snack and dinnertime, after a morning injection of intermediate insulin, a mixture of carbohydrate and protein, such as low-fat yogurt or crackers and cheese, is recommended.

Carbohydrates provide energy to meet the body's more immediate needs. The addition of protein to the snack helps sustain the blood glucose levels for a longer period, slowing gastric emptying. This can be important in a bedtime snacking plan.

### Fiber

Dietary fiber is present in all fruits and vegetables. It is the structural component of plant tissue that cannot be digested by human enzymes. There are two types of dietary fiber: soluble and insoluble. Each functions differently in the body.

Insoluble fiber is found in bran cereals, whole-grain breads, whole fruits, and vegetables. It is called insoluble because it does not dissolve in water. This type of fiber adds bulk to the diet and speeds passage of foods through the intestines. Its utility in preventing or alleviating constipation is due to the laxative effect of the more rapid passage of food through the digestive tract.

Soluble fiber, which is found in oats, dried beans, whole fruits, and vegetables, is so named because it dissolves in water to form a gummy gel. This gel slows the passage of food through the digestive tract. Recent studies have also shown that soluble fiber may also be useful in lowering blood cholesterol levels.

Most Americans consume about 10 to 20 grams of dietary fiber per day. However, researchers recommend increasing this to 20 to 35 grams. This dietary change should be made gradually, though, because a sudden increase in fiber can result in increased flatulence (gas) and cramping. When you decide to increase your fiber, be sure you also drink more fluids. The fluids help increase the intestinal bulk, resulting in softer, larger stools, which are more comfortable to eliminate.

## Vegetarianism

A vegetarian diet low in fat and high in fiber may be beneficial in lowering the risk of heart disease while still meeting caloric, protein, vitamin, and mineral requirements.

If you are interested in trying a vegetarian plan, be sure you slowly increase the fiber content of your diet to avoid bloating and cramping. Foods high in fiber may raise the blood sugar more slowly, so less insulin may be required for the same amount of carbohydrate at meal times.

Generally, a vegetarian meal is higher in carbohydrate content than a nonvegetarian meal. With the higher carbohydrate content relative to protein and fat, postmeal blood glucose levels may be higher than desired even though premeal blood sugars are within target range.

You may find it necessary to divide the meal into smaller meals and larger snacks so you consume adequate calories while minimizing the glucose fluctuations after meals.

## Weight gain and intensive therapy

Weight gain is a common complaint of people undertaking intensive diabetes therapy. Explanations for this gain include improved caloric efficiency (using all the calories you take in and not losing them in the urine), experimentation with new foods, increased frequency of hypoglycemic reactions that require extra food, and larger meals.

Theoretically, consuming only an extra 25 calories per day can result in a 3-pound weight gain in a year! Remember, with rapid improvement in diabetes control, you may have temporary fluid retention that may make you think you have gained even more weight.

Therefore, you must pay careful attention to the meal plan and how it balances with the other factors in your diabetes control. Weight gain does *not* have to occur with intensive insulin therapy, but the chances are much greater if you do not develop and follow a careful meal plan.

One pitfall when using intensive diabetes therapy is that insulin adjustment makes overeating tempting. Insulin can be increased to cover extra food or desserts. Taking more food and more insulin may maintain desirable glucose levels, but it also increases the number of calories that will be stored as fat, rather than being lost in the urine!

Therefore, you cannot ignore the total calories consumed, even though you know how to adapt your insulin for extra food intake and maintain good glucose control. Be aware of the caloric content of a food item to help prevent weight gain. Fat, especially, must be watched, because calories from fat are more efficiently converted to fat stores than are calories from protein or carbohydrate.

### Carbohydrate counting

The basic meal plan is designed to account for your caloric needs, meal times, and meal size preferences based on an estimate of basic metabolic needs. However, sometimes you may want more or less food at meal and snack times. Or you may just want to try some new foods.

Since carbohydrate is the food component that affects blood sugar levels the most, the amounts and types of carbohydrate ideally should be consistent for a specific insulin dose. Theoretically, the more carbohydrate consumed at a meal, the higher the dose of regular insulin needed. Conversely, less insulin is needed for less carbohydrate.

Use your meal plan as a starting point for deriving a ratio of insulin-to-carbohydrate meal load. By keeping records of food eaten, insulin taken, and postmeal blood glucose values you will be able to calculate how much regular insulin your body requires for carbo-hydrates taken in a specific meal.

To get this information, just add the total number of grams of carbohydrate eaten at the specific meal and divide this number by the units of premeal regular insulin. This ratio is often found to be about 1 to 2 units insulin for each 15 grams of carbohydrate. Your postmeal blood glucose will tell you whether the regular insulin taken before the meal was sufficient to bring your blood glucose back into a desirable range.

Of course, for this approach to allow successful insulin dose adjustments, you need to accurately estimate the approximate carbohydrate content of the meal you are about to eat *before* eating it. Spur-of-the-moment overindulging will foul things up, for sure!

Estimating the carbohydrate content is easier when you know the approximate carbohydrate composition of the food groups. You can obtain exchange lists that provide general approximations of carbohydrate content from the American Diabetes Association or from the Joslin Diabetes Center. Or you can purchase a pocket carbohydrate counting guide at many bookstores.

| Food group | Carbohydrate per serving |
|------------|--------------------------|
| Bread | 15 gm |
| Fruit | 15 gm |
| Vegetable | 5 gm |
| Milk | 12 gm |
| Meat | 0 gm |
| Fat | 0 gm |

Using carbohydrate counting, you place greater emphasis on the carbohydrate content of a whole meal, rather than on the individual food group components (1 fruit, 2 breads, 2 meats, and the like). One serving from the fruit group contributes 15 grams of carbohydrate, the same amount as one serving from the bread group.

To effectively make such estimates, become familiar with portion sizes, especially in the carbohydrate-containing food groups. This will allow more accurate estimations of the insulin dose adjustments needed to cover a given meal.

For example, you are planning to eat this meal:

| *Sandwich* | *Carbohydrate (grams)* |
|------------|------------------------|
| 2 slices of bread | 30 |
| 2 ounces of turkey | 0 |
| 1 tablespoon mayonnaise | 0 |
| 1 medium apple | 15 |
| 8 ounces low-fat milk | 12 |
| 4 ounces low-fat sugarfree yogurt | 15 |
| Total carbohydrate content: | 72 grams |

Let's assume your premeal insulin dose according to your algorithm is set for a carbohydrate content of 50 grams. Because the meal contains 72 grams of carbohydrate, you probably will need 1 to 2 extra units of regular insulin to keep blood sugars within target range.

Records of the carbohydrate content of meals, premeal insulin doses, and blood glucose levels before and after meals will help you define your own carbohydrate-insulin ratio. Of course, other factors such as exercise and the time interval between insulin injection and the actual meal time also must be taken into consideration. In addition, some people find they need more regular insulin to cover the carbohydrate in their breakfast.

## Problem-solving with diet

It is nearly a knee-jerk response among those of us caring for people with diabetes, and people with diabetes themselves, to adjust the insulin dose when something is not right with blood sugar control. Yet, so many other factors contribute to diabetes control, that doing so may just frustrate you while not really solving the problem.

Often, once your insulin program is well adapted to your metabolic needs, we stop changing doses when problems arise and look for other factors. Food certainly is at the top of that list!

Listed below are some problems people using intensive diabetes therapy often encounter and some suggestions for adjusting the diet to solve them.

### High postmeal blood glucose, with levels on target by the next premeal test

Frequently, high post-meal blood glucose levels may result in high glycohemoglobin levels in individuals who are getting "good" test results before meals, emphasizing the need to pay attention to the test made one and a half to two hours after a meal.

The fat and carbohydrate content of a meal affect the postmeal glucose levels. High fat meals, such as pizza or a hamburger and french fries, can result in high postmeal blood glucose levels for up to 5 hours after the meal.

Similarly, very large amounts of carbohydrate may cause high glucose values after meals. Separating out some of the carbohydrate from a meal into a later snack will prevent this problem, which may be seen with vegetarian meal plans. The size of the carbohydrate-heavy meals needs to be reduced in favor of between-meal snacks.

### Low blood glucose levels at the crisscross of two insulins' action curves

When taking multiple insulin injections throughout the day, you will often find periods when one insulin's action is waning as another's is building toward its peak. An example is the late morning if you use a morning mixed dose of regular plus an intermediate insulin. The regular insulin action is subsiding, while the intermediate insulin is increasing its effect. If hypoglycemic reactions occur at this time, it is often difficult to determine which insulin is the most to blame and even more difficult to arrive at a satisfactory solution. Diet adjustments may help.

If the time between meals is great, blood glucose levels are more likely to drop too low during the interval. Of course, if the postmeal blood glucose levels are low as well, the insulin dose can be reduced. However, you may need a between-meal snack to prevent a drop during the between-meal period if reducing the actual insulin doses would create high sugars at other times.

Adding or increasing the size of this snack may allow you to prevent the hypoglycemic reactions without having to decrease either insulin dose. Adding snacks can increase caloric intake, however. So, if you don't want to gain weight, you may need to subtract food for the snack from some other meal.

Reducing total food intake to lose weight without properly adjusting your insulin doses can also create this situation. If you eat less food, you should require less insulin. Test your blood frequently during any period of dieting to avoid having to "eat up to an insulin dose" and defeating your efforts at weight loss.

### High fasting sugars with low middle-of-the-night (3 A.M.) sugars

There are many reasons for high fasting blood sugar levels. The pattern of a low blood sugar at 3 A.M. and a high fasting value suggests that a nocturnal reaction has resulted in a rebound high sugar before your breakfast.

You may need to add or increase the size of a bedtime snack. Examine the content of this snack. Does it contain enough protein to prolong its effect through the night, or is it all carbohydrate? Are you eating it too early, so the effect is gone by the time the insulin peaks at 3 A.M? And don't forget the "lag effect" from exercise. Activity in the evening—a formal exercise program or *any* activity—can cause glucose levels to drop some hours later. A larger bedtime snack may be helpful in preventing this drop. Ideally, snacks at bedtime should include at least one starch and one lean meat.

Finally, if you really want to avoid any weight gain, especially if you are already eating a bedtime snack at the proper time and with the proper constituents, you may have to consider reducing the insulin dose.

### Treating hypoglycemia reactions

Hypoglycemic reactions are more common with intensive insulin therapy as blood sugars are closer to normal, with less "margin of error." Early warning symptoms of hypoglycemia—shakiness, nervousness, and sweating—should be confirmed with a blood sugar test and treated immediately to prevent development of the more serious symptoms of confusion, disorientation, and unconsciousness.

With the first suggestion of hypoglycemia, test your blood sugar. If it is below the target levels you and your health team have agreed upon, eat a 15-gram dose of a fast-acting carbohydrate, such as sugar itself or glucose tablets. These do not contain fat or protein to slow down glucose absorption. If the symptoms are still present 15 to 20 minutes later or if your blood glucose is still low, take a second dose of fast-acting carbohydrate.

If the hypoglycemic reaction occurred no more than an hour before a scheduled meal or snack, eat the meal or snack after treatment. If the meal or snack is scheduled to be eaten more than an hour later, an additional snack containing a slow-acting carbohydrate plus protein will help sustain your glucose level until then.

Weight-conscious individuals can subtract these calories from the next meal and adjust their insulin dose accordingly. However, prudence in preventing the reactions is the best way to avoid this problem!

Always review the events preceding the reaction and try to determine why it occurred.
- Did you skip or delay a meal or snack?
- Were you more active without increasing your food or decreasing insulin dose?
- Did you take too much insulin?

Also, blood sugar levels may rise after the reaction from the rebound phenomenon, but frequently much of this rise is caused by overtreating the reaction. Pay close attention to the amount of food you use to treat reactions. With experience, you will take just enough and not too much. Be sure that the snack's content is correct, as well. Treatment with slow-acting carbohydrates or with foods containing protein or fat may delay the effect of that treatment, and you may need additional food.

## Erratic blood sugars

People using intensive diabetes therapy often have glucose logs that show values "all over the place." Where do you start solving this frustrating problem?

Many factors can influence blood sugar control—timing, size and composition of meals, activity, and insulin doses, to name the major ones. With so many variables to juggle, it's no wonder that test results at times can become erratic and show no pattern. Sorting out the factors is a challenge, but the usual approach is to "get back to basics." Identify all of the variables and begin to make an effort to maintain a more regular schedule of eating and exercising.

From the meal planning standpoint, this means keeping the time and spacing of meals consistent for several days. Note how much carbohydrate you eat at meals and, ideally, keep it constant.

Minimize variability in activity both to fix that variable and also to prevent the need for additional snacking during this control period. Exercise a set amount and at a fixed time—or even suspend exercise altogether—until the patterns can be smoothed out.

## Sick days

A full discussion on how to manage sick days can be found in Chapters 7 and 11, but from the meal planning standpoint, keep these issues in mind. Insulin is still required when you are ill, yet there are times when it is difficult to keep food down or to eat or drink as usual. This can make taking insulin problematic or dangerous. Overall, your goal is to take in adequate fluids and to maintain blood glucose control as much as possible.

When eating is difficult, try salty fluids such as broth, consomme, or tomato juice, if tolerated, to help maintain your fluid level. Include good sources of potassium, such as Gatorade® or orange juice. Rotate calorie-containing fluids with noncaloric beverages and salty broths to help maintain fluid and blood sugar levels. This is even more important if any vomiting or diarrhea has occurred, which can cause you to lose sodium, potassium, and fluid.

For a sick day eating guide, your meal plan is converted to easy-to-eat-or-drink carbohydrate sources. Your goal is to try to keep the amount of carbohydrate constant, since this is the component of the

| Converting a meal plan for a sick day | | |
|---|---|---|
| Meal plan | Sample menu for sick day | Carbohydrate (grams) |
| **Dinner, 6 P.M.** | | |
| 2 vegetable | 3 ounces gingerale | 10 |
| 1 fruit | 1/2 cup unsweetened applesauce | 15 |
| 2 bread | 1/2 cup sherbet | 30 |
| 4 meat | No substitution necessary | 0 |
| 1 fat | No substitution necessary | 0 |
| **Snack, 9 P.M.** | | |
| 1 bread | 1 popsicle, 3 ounces | 15 |
| 1 meat | No substitution necessary | 0 |
| **Total carbo-hydrate: 70 gm** | | **70 gm** |

diet that will affect blood sugar levels the most. The food is spread throughout the day as small meals, which you may tolerate better than larger meals.

If you have nausea, try clear liquids such as regular (sugar-containing) gelatin, soda, broth, and apple juice. You may tolerate these better than than heavier or creamier items. Foods that contain more sugar than usually recommended can be used on a sick day when used in small amounts.

## Alcohol

While alcohol contains no carbohydrate, protein, or fat and has no nutritional value, it does provide calories—7 calories per gram, in fact! Alcohol is absorbed from the stomach and transported to the liver where it is metabolized.

The liver also stores glucose in the form of glycogen, but when it is busy metabolizing alcohol, it cannot release glucose as well as it should if the blood glucose level falls too low. Therefore, if you wish to consume alcoholic beverages, you need to eat something along with the alcohol to slow its absorption.

Certain alcoholic beverages such as sweet wines, cordials, and liqueurs contain large amounts of carbohydrate that can cause blood sugar elevations. Beverages such as dry wines, light beer, or hard liquors contain less sugar and carbohydrate, and are preferable.

Light beer is preferable to regular beer because light has less carbohydrate. Alcohol-free beers have even less. An 8-ounce glass of regular beer can contain as much carbohydrate as a slice of bread. If you choose a hard liquor, mix 1 ounce with water, ice, diet soda, or a sugar-free mixer. Cocktails prepared in this way contain about 85 calories.

The traditional prohibition against alcohol consumption for people with diabetes has been liberalized somewhat. However, moderation is important for everyone, *especially* if you have diabetes. Alcohol should only be used when blood sugars are in good control.

The effects of alcohol on people using intensive diabetes therapy are no different than for those on conventional therapies. However, because of the high goals and close scrutiny of glucose levels in intensive therapy, alcohol can have a greater effect on management. A thorough understanding of the effects of alcohol on your diabetes is essential for maintaining good glucose levels.

## Glycemic index

Although we have discussed the role of carbohydrate counting in adjusting insulin in intensive insulin therapy, it's worth noting that a given amount of carbohydrate may not always have the same effect on your blood glucose levels.

Some thought to this "glycemic index concept" may help you troubleshoot occasional problems in diabetes control.

The glycemic index concept was devised to explain apparent differences in the blood glucose responses between apparently similar amounts of carbohydrate. To develop the glycemic index, a slice of white bread was used as a reference food. The change in blood glucose from before to after the bread was eaten was designated as standard and assigned a value of 100.

Effects of other foods were then compared with those of the slice of white bread. Ice cream, for example, with a surprisingly slow glycemic response, had a value of 52, while instant potatoes with a more rapid response had a value of 116. Kidney beans had a value of 54.

Clearly, if ice cream has a value of only 52, many factors affect the glycemic index. Protein and fat slow gastric emptying and result in a lower glycemic index. Liquids are absorbed more rapidly than solids. Water-soluble fibers delay gastric emptying, which reduces the glycemic response.

By keeping records of your own response to different carbohydrate in meals, you can determine your own glycemic index, which will help you understand variations in your postmeal blood glucose.

Keep in mind, too, that the glycemic index does not take calories into consideration. For example, half a cup of ice cream has a lower glycemic response (about half) than half a cup of instant mashed potatoes. But don't replace the potatoes with two scoops of vanilla too fast. Ice cream contains *four times* the calories and *200 times* the fat!

Keep in mind, however, that when eating a mixed meal—a customary meal with various food types—the differences in glycemic response of various carbohydrates disappear. Protein and fat mixed in with carbohydrates in your meal work to dilute the effect of any single carbohydrate. For this reason, you can incorporate small amounts of sugar (1 to 2 teaspoons) into a meal without disturbing your blood glucose control. What matters is the amount of total carbohydrate in your meals, because your body will convert any type of carbohydrate into sugar at about the same rate.

## Summary

It has become increasingly obvious to health care professionals that the one factor likely to dictate whether you will be successful or not in treatment goals is how well you understand and follow your meal plan. Without close attention, no intensive insulin therapy is likely to succeed.

While much of this book discusses insulin doses and their adjustment, never forget your meal plan. Now that you understand how food can affect intensive insulin therapy, you may be surprised at how often you will recognize factors that have been affecting your diabetes control.

The old saying "you are what you eat" can truly be adapted to apply to an intensive insulin therapy program by saying "it is what you eat!"

# Chapter Six

# Using Multiple Daily Insulin Injections

## What's this section about?

■ Exactly what are your options with injections?

■ What about an ultralente program?

Intensifying someone's diabetes therapy is often a stepwise process. The first step is to modify a conventional program into an "intensified conventional" regimen. The second step is into true intensive therapy and uses more complex, physiologic multiple daily injection (MDI) programs. The next step is to use continuous subcutaneous insulin infusion (CSII, the pumps).

These programs have already been referred to in earlier sections. But this chapter presents the injected insulin treatment programs in detail, to help you with self-management and to assist you if you are considering intensive diabetes therapy and want details about the different programs available.

We focus on the most frequently used programs, with references to some of the less common variations. The list may not include every reasonable or possible combination, but it provides specifics about a variety of programs that will be useful to most people choosing injected intensified conventional and intensive diabetes therapies.

Your choice of program is determined by your own needs, both in adapting therapy to your schedule and in matching it to your insulin requirements. If everyone were the same, this chapter would contain only one program. Since everyone is different, you have a choice.

## Intensified conventional programs

> **We do not recommend beginning any of the treatment programs discussed in this book without guidance from a physician.**

*General considerations.* The "split-mix" is the cornerstone of conventional treatment of type I diabetes and is the basis of the intensified conventional treatment approaches. Traditionally, there have been two major variations of the split mix:

1. A mixture of regular and intermediate insulin (NPH or lente) before breakfast, and a mixture of regular and intermediate insulin before supper.
2. A mixture of regular and intermediate insulin before breakfast, and intermediate at bedtime.

Recently, with the more precisely timed but shorter acting human insulins, conventional therapies have also included a three-injection variation:

3. Regular and intermediate insulin before breakfast, regular insulin before supper, and intermediate insulin at bedtime.

To qualify as an intensive diabetes therapy program, an algorithm must be designed with adjustments for blood glucose tests at least *three* times daily. Programs with one or two daily dose adjustments are considered "intensified conventional" therapies. Yet, in designing programs, the differences between intensified conventional therapies and true intensive therapies sometimes become blurred.

Intensified conventional programs use insulin doses that peak at significant points during the day, usually coinciding with meals. No single insulin dose provides the basal insulin supply; the overlapping action of different peaking doses serves this purpose.

### Advantages and disadvantages

There are theoretical advantages and disadvantages to the use of intensified conventional therapy. One advantage is the obvious simplicity of these programs compared with the more complex intensive therapies. Also, peaking intermediate insulin may be more effective than the smoother patterns of basal insulin, ultralente, or a pump in keeping or bringing blood glucose levels down in patients with significant insulin resistance. This is especially true at night; peaking insulin toward the end of the sleep cycle can be effective for people with high fasting blood glucose levels caused by a prominent dawn phenomenon.

Another advantage is that insulins that peak and wane allow for scheduled dips when less insulin is needed, such as during or after exercise.

However, some of these advantages may also be disadvantages. Insulins peak at specified times and last for specified durations. If your schedule doesn't quite fit the pharmacological properties of the insulin, you may have problems coordinating insulin action with real life. Snacks, changes in schedule or insulin type, and occasional compromises in control may be necessary.

For example, one variation of the two–injection split-mix program uses ultralente instead of intermediate insulin at suppertime in an attempt to spread the insulin effect over a longer time. However, this compromises the benefit of the intermediate insulin's strong peak, because ultralente's peak is much less prominent and effective than that of NPH or lente.

Another problem is that intermediate insulin peaks 8 hours after injection, rather than 3 to 4 hours later as with regular insulin. With an intensive program using regular insulin, the regular insulin works over a shorter time, allowing more opportunities during the day for adjustments. Intermediate insulin essentially acts over a third to half of the day, and it may be difficult to predict insulin needs 8 hours in advance. Once you have taken intermediate insulin, you are less able to adapt for changes in your insulin needs, say, 4 hours later.

Also, onset, peak, and duration of action for intermediate insulins are less predictable than for regular insulin. The newer human insulins may be more predictable than animal insulins. Unless their shorter duration is a problem, human insulins are usually preferred for intensive therapy.

To compensate for the imprecision of intermediate insulins, you can adjust the dosing schedule or use regular insulin at other times. This allows a reduced dose of the intermediate insulin. For example, you take regular insulin at lunchtime, reducing your morning intermediate dose. You expect that the intermediate insulin, although still peaking, will act like a basal dose with a lower peak. The regular insulin is used to respond to the glucose level and accommodate for eating and activity.

## Specific intensified conventional programs

### • Standard split-mix (regular plus intermediate before breakfast and again before supper)

This program allows two daily dosing decisions—one at breakfast and one at suppertime. The expectation that the morning intermediate insulin will effectively cover the afternoon insulin requirements can cause problems. Because this program occasionally has difficulty with proper intermediate insulin coverage during the day, an alternative scale using less morning intermediate, which acts as a basal insulin, plus prelunch regular may be more effective. (This program of three regular insulin injections qualifies as intensive therapy.)

People who take their injection early in the morning have other problems with the standard split-mix. There are two possible times during the day when they are prone to hypoglycemia. One is midmorning, especially if the interval between breakfast and lunch is great (5 or 6 hours). The crisscrossing effect of the waning regular and the sizeable intermediate insulin dose building to its peak may cause hypoglycemia, and prevention often requires midmorning snacks.

The other problem time is midafternoon, when early morning intermediate insulin is peaking. This is not the time that many people eat dinner! Another snack is often necessary, which may boost the glucose level later in the afternoon as the intermediate insulin passes its peak and begins to diminish. This often results in the dinnertime glucose level being too high. Increasing the morning insulin increases the chance of worse midafternoon hypoglycemia, without lowering the presupper glucose levels.

A similar problem exists at night. The presupper intermediate insulin peaks during the middle of the night (2 to 3 A.M.) when less insulin is required, and its effect is waning by 4 or 5 A.M., when more insulin is needed because of the dawn phenomenon.

Therefore, the two-injection split-mix program should be used only as intensified conventional therapy for people who can't use or don't want the three-injection variety (described below) or true intensive therapy. An algorithm is used for the morning and presupper regular insulin doses to allow some flexibility. However, use of these programs requires significant compromises.

### • Regular plus intermediate insulin before breakfast, regular before supper, intermediate (and regular insulin if necessary) at bedtime

This program is a significant variation on the standard split-mix. It is commonly used with fixed doses as conventional diabetes treatment, as well as with variable doses of regular insulin as an intensified conventional therapy.

Giving the second injection of intermediate insulin at bedtime compensates for the overnight timing problem; the insulin peaks just as the dawn phenomenon is having its effect. It is most useful for people whose morning injection is late enough so the intermediate insulin peak time and duration of action are timed properly.

This program does not include a noontime dosing decision point unless one is added, but doing so would lead to four daily injections and the program would then resemble the premeal regular and bedtime intermediate intensive program described later in this chapter.

As described here, this program might allow three decision points for the use of regular insulin: breakfast, supper, and bedtime, although regular insulin should not be given at bedtime unless the glucose level is quite high. Of course, for those prone to overindulge at the dinner table, this may be more often than not!

The variant of this program that substitutes ultralente insulin for the breakfast intermediate insulin is useful for people who eat an early breakfast and late supper and need a longer insulin duration than that of intermediate insulin. However, this variation usually requires a prelunch injection of regular as well, because the coverage of the poorly peaking ultralente usually is not sufficient to cover lunch and afternoon requirements.

High fasting blood glucose levels with this modified split-mix program usually can be handled fairly easily. Once you rule out nocturnal hypoglycemia by occasionally testing in the middle of the night, you can increase the bedtime intermediate insulin. This usually corrects the problem. Nevertheless, if more than 8 or 9 hours elapse between bedtime and arising, the insulin action wanes before the time of the dawn phenomenon.

It is possible that the blood glucose is on an upswing right at bedtime. The suppertime regular has run out, and the bedtime intermediate has not yet started to work. Bedtime regular might provide catch-up. But more regular insulin at suppertime often corrects this problem. Some people have tried a small dose of intermediate insulin with the suppertime regular to help bridge this gap.

High sugars during the day are covered with more of the appropriate insulin or by adding lunchtime regular, as outlined previously. Problematic hypoglycemia with this program often requires a reduction of the regular insulin and an increase in the NPH, but you might consider using an ultralente program (discussed later), which may be more stabilizing.

## Variations

Variations of this basic intensified conventional program are often used to overcome the shortcomings of this program. Some of these variations bring this program quite close to a true intensive therapy regimen.

### • Regular plus intermediate insulin before breakfast, regular plus ultralente insulin before supper

From an insulin-action standpoint, this is a two-injection variant of the above program for people who do not want to take three daily injections, but have difficulty with the earlier peak and shorter duration of presupper intermediate insulin. It is not a true three-injection intensive insulin therapy, and is most effective when the morning injection is taken late enough so the intermediate insulin peak and its duration of action in the afternoon coincides with supper.

When compared with suppertime intermediate insulin, timing of the overnight ultralente peak may be more effectively coordinated with the dawn phenomenon. However, ultralente's peak is less pronounced. Also, unit for unit, it may be less effective than intermediate insulin. Ultralente may also last well into the midmorning period the next day and overlap with the morning regular insulin action.

### • Regular plus intermediate insulin before breakfast, regular insulin before lunch, and regular plus ultralente insulin before supper

This is a combination of the previous program plus a reduced morning intermediate insulin dose and prelunch regular. If timed correctly, it is effective for those who eat later breakfasts and earlier suppers, and who can be adequately treated overnight with the presupper ultralente. It allows three decision points for regular insulin dose adjustment and technically qualifies as an intensive program.

High fasting glucose levels are not uncommon with this program because ultralente is less effective against the dawn phenomenon. Rule out hypoglycemia at 2 to 3 A.M., and then increase the suppertime ultralente if necessary. Adjust the timing of the injection if the ultralente peaks at a time other than the end of the sleep cycle.

Ultimately, if these maneuvers are not helpful, a program using bedtime intermediate insulin or even a pump with an alternate basal dose may be needed. The approach to high daytime glucose levels with this insulin pattern has already been discussed (see page 95).

### • Regular plus ultralente insulin before breakfast, regular insulin at lunchtime, and regular plus intermediate insulin before supper

This program is the opposite of the one discussed above, with timing the major difference. Again, it technically qualifies as intensive therapy.

If you arise early and have a long span between breakfast and supper, the longer-acting ultralente in the morning may be more effective as a basal-type insulin dose. With a blunted peak, a prelunch regular insulin dosing scale is almost always needed.

If you eat dinner late enough, timing of the presupper intermediate insulin controls the glucose levels through the night. (If not and ultralente is substituted at night as well, the program becomes a dual ultralente program, discussed later in this chapter.)

Adjustments for high fasting glucose levels are the same here as for any program using suppertime intermediate insulin. If the insulin peaks too early, causing reactions and rebounds, or does not last long enough, or both, you may need to change to ultralente or a program using bedtime intermediate insulin. High glucose levels during the day require adjustments similar to those listed previously.

## Multidose regular intensive diabetes therapy

The hallmark of programs using multiple doses of regular insulin is the predominant reliance on this rapid acting insulin between meals. The levels of insulin in the blood rise and fall during the day with the peaks and valleys of the regular insulin action. During the night, blood glucose control is maintained by either twice-daily ultralente or NPH or lente insulin at bedtime.

The choice between ultralente and NPH or lente for nocturnal control has been discussed previously. An advantage of ultralente programs is that they might allow a reduction in the number of injections from four per day to three.

Occasionally, the smoother ultralente action is useful if nocturnal hypoglycemia is a problem. Bedtime intermediate allows another decision point during the day and tends to be more effective for people with fasting hyperglycemia caused by the dawn phenomenon.

## Premeal regular and bedtime intermediate insulin

These programs use only premeal regular insulin during the day. Overlapping regular insulin provides some basal effect. Bedtime intermediate insulin provides nighttime coverage.

An advantage of this multidose regular program is that primary control for the upcoming time period rests with the short-acting regular dose. There is minimal overlap from other insulins. Thus, you have complete control over insulin levels if you need this precision or the ability to make last minute decisions more accurately.

For example, if you exercise vigorously and have had difficulty with hypoglycemia either during exercise or afterward due to lag effect, you could coordinate your insulin and exercise to allow the insulin level to drop quite low when needed.

There are disadvantages, too. If you have long days, with an early breakfast and late supper, you may have long intervals between regular insulin doses. The regular insulin may run out before the next dose is given. Without a basal insulin acting during this time, the low insulin level can result in rising blood glucose levels. Adding a small morning dose of intermediate or ultralente to provide some basal effect may help cover these intervals.

Glucose levels controlled by rising and falling regular insulin levels may provide an advantage if you like or need complete control from your short-acting insulin. However, for people with very unstable diabetes, extreme ups and downs of the insulin level can perpetuate instability. A program that has some basal insulin effect during the day might be preferable for these individuals.

Making insulin dose adjustments in a premeal regular and bedtime intermediate insulin program is, in some ways, simpler than with other programs. Usually there is only one insulin with any significant action during a given period. If the sugar is high, raise that dose, if it is low, lower that dose!

Yet, such simplicity doesn't always lead to the correct solution. For example, increasing the premeal dose might not be the best solution for a high postmeal glucose that is back to normal or even low before the next meal. With regular insulin alone, it usually isn't possible to increase the effect early in its action curve and decrease it later on.

If the premeal glucose level before that first meal was high, increasing the previous insulin dose might help. On the other hand, you might try increasing the time between the injection and the meal or changing the content of the meal to prevent a rise in glucose.

There is an old adage about diabetes treatment: "As you start the day, so goes the day." In other words, if you start the day with a glucose level on target, the rest of the day is more likely to remain on target. Why? Even the best designed adjustment programs tend to be more effective at *maintaining* steady blood glucose levels than at bringing them down. There's always the risk of over- or undershooting.

This concern is especially true for this type of multidose regular insulin program. Therefore, what happens to glucose levels overnight is quite important. There is no substitute for frequent nocturnal monitoring and close attention to patterns.

Adjustment of the overnight insulin action by altering the bedtime intermediate insulin has been discussed with previous programs and the same principles apply here.

### • Programs using premeal regular plus ultralente as a basal insulin supply

Ultralente, available for many years, had fallen into disfavor because of its unpredictable peak time and duration of action. With intensive diabetes therapy, however, ultralente has been born again!

Ultralente provides a longer duration of action than intermediate insulins and, when given regularly in moderate quantities, provides an effective basal insulin supply to supplement premeal regular insulin doses.

*Frequency of ultralente dose*—Most people give ultralente before breakfast and before supper. This spreads the doses 10 to 14 hours apart, which fairly effectively provides a basal insulin supply. One injection a day tends to produce more of a peaking effect, especially with human ultralente. Some people have advocated giving ultralente before all three meals, but this is probably spreading it out more than necessary.

*Mixing ultralente with regular insulin*—Clearly, if ultralente could be mixed with regular insulin, you could use this program with three injections per day. But some experts recommend that these insulins not be mixed, resulting in the need for five daily injections. Does it make a difference? The answer is . . . maybe!

Zinc is used in the manufacture of ultralente to help it last as long as it does. When ultralente is mixed with regular insulin, some of the regular combines with the zinc, resulting in prolonged regular insulin action. This can make the regular insulin less effective in the period immediately after eating.

How much regular insulin binds in this manner is increased by two factors: a great excess of ultralente (and thus, zinc) over regular in the syringe promotes more combining and the longer the insulins remain mixed in the same syringe, the more regular combines with zinc.

So mixing these two insulins does make a difference. But does this difference really affect the treatment of your diabetes? Well, maybe!

To decide, think about the design of an ultralente program. Your health care team estimates starting doses for ultralente and the regular algorithm. You use these doses while keeping careful records and then adjust the doses to fit your needs. You might discover that you need more regular insulin effect and less ultralente effect, possibly because more of the regular insulin you mix in the syringe acts longer. You can then adjust your program to use less ultralente and more regular. A simple solution! Indeed, this is often what happens. Then you can maintain an ultralente program with three, rather than five, daily injections.

What have you sacrificed by doing this? You have lost some of the "kick" from the rapid-acting regular insulin. Whether this is a serious problem for you depends on your therapy goals. If you have achieved goals such as smoothing out your control, compensating for scheduling, activity, or eating, and improving your glycohemoglobin but are unhappy about using five daily injections, then giving separate injections is not necessary.

However, if you have been unable to reach your goals or want the lowest glycohemoglobin safely achievable and are willing to take five daily injections, then you should consider splitting up the regular and ultralente. First, document your after-meal glucose levels and glycohemoglobin, then make the change to split ultralente and regular, keeping other variables constant. After a few months, you can decide whether the change in after-meal glucose levels and glycohemoglobin justifies giving regular and ultralente separately.

Before human ultralente was available, ultralente insulin had diffuse peaks and a long duration of action. Given either once a day or in two equal doses, it provided a smooth basal effect. Since it was effectively peakless, however, it provided poor coverage for the dawn phenomenon.

Now, with human ultralente's more obvious and predictable peaks, more people are successfully adjusting the ratio between the two ultralente doses. Giving more ultralente at suppertime than in the morning covers the dawn phenomenon better. Conversely, if you eat more of your daily food at suppertime, you may benefit from more ultralente in the morning. Ratio adjustments must be individualized, but many people benefit from unequal doses.

Insulin doses must be tailored to individual needs, of course. Yet, for very few people is there *one* insulin program that is *clearly* the best. There can be many approaches that fill your needs.

Nevertheless, certain multiple daily injection programs are used more often because of some clear advantages. One plan uses the ratio between ultralente and regular, usually a ratio of *about* 50 /50. (Most people vary from 40/60 to 60/40.) Half of the daily insulin is ultralente and half is regular, divided among the various doses.

One advantage of this plan is that the usual dose adjustments (generally increments of 1 unit or so) are a reasonable percent of your total daily dose to work effectively. If your morning insulin dose for a glucose level of 100 to 150 mg/dl is only 2 units of regular with 36 units of ultralente, even minimal regular dose adjustments would involve too large a percent of the total.

Not everyone needs a 50/50 ratio. If you are way off, and your program is not going well, it may be worth trying a different ratio to see if things get better.

## Starting an ultralente program

The following are rough guidelines to show how you and your health care team may approach an ultralente program.

The total daily insulin dose is calculated as 0.5 units of insulin per kilogram of actual body weight. Half of this total is given as ultralente, half before breakfast and half before supper. The other half of the daily total is given as regular insulin.

An algorithm is designed so 40 percent of half the daily dose is given as regular insulin before breakfast, with 30 percent each before lunch and before supper. Regular doses are stepped up for glucose levels above normal and stepped down for lower levels.

Once the program is begun, glucose levels must be recorded carefully. Unless glucose levels are dangerously high or low, achieving appropriate fasting glucose levels should be the first target. These levels are controlled primarily by the ultralente.

If your glucose levels are generally high, consider the total ultralente dose as affecting the fasting glucose level, and increase both your breakfast and supper quantities equally, one unit at a time. If daytime values begin to approach the low 100 mg/dl range while the fasting values are still too high, increase the suppertime ultralente.

When the fasting glucose levels are at or close to the target range, begin adjusting the regular insulin. (A discussion of adjustments of regular insulin is included in Chapter 4.)

## Summary

Throughout this book, we discuss the philosophy of intensive diabetes therapy and provide adjustment guidelines for various programs. Yet, like the programs themselves, specific adjustments must be individualized for both the person with diabetes and the health care team.

Here the art of medicine comes in to play. If you asked 10 artists to paint the same vista, the result would be 10 totally different paintings. Similarly, giving 10 different intensive diabetes teams one patient to work with can result in 10 different treatment approaches.

Therefore, guidelines in this chapter on MDI programs should not be viewed as a "color-by-numbers" approach to painting an intensive diabetes program. Rather, think of them as instructions on how to use the paints! You and your treatment team are the artists who will turn the blank canvas into a picture of a treatment that works for you!

# Using Insulin Pumps

Use of continuous subcutaneous insulin infusion (CSII) therapy with an insulin infusion device (pump) is usually the next step in intensity after multiple daily injection programs. Pump use requires even more self-care and attention than MDI. It is a more complex insulin delivery system than a simple syringe; with the constant infusion of only short-acting regular insulin, consequences of too much or too little insulin occur rapidly and with little warning. The decision to embark on pump therapy should not be taken lightly. Only begin a pump therapy program if you have access to a treatment team skilled in working with many pump therapy patients.

Pump therapy can provide better control than other methods of intensive therapy. But this "better" therapy requires more motivation, dexterity, judgment, psychological stability, and self-management efforts and skills than other methods of intensive therapy. It also is expensive.

While the $4,000 cost (in 1994 dollars) of the pumps may be partially covered by health insurance (many cover only 80 percent), the supplies, including insulin, syringes, catheters, and dressings, may run $25 to $30 a week, and insurance coverage may vary.

## Risks with pumps

Use of an insulin infusion pump poses risks that you *must* understand and be willing to accept—and also be willing to work to prevent. Some are minor, some are major. Only begin a pump program under the supervision of a physician and a health care team skilled in pump therapy.

Pumps infuse insulin through a needle inserted into the skin. Complications can include inflammation, infection, or localized reactions at the needle insertion site. When you inject insulin by syringe, you rotate sites so each site is only used every few weeks. Because catheter insertion sites have insulin infusing constantly over a two-day period, nodules may form at the insertion sites from local skin reactions to insulin. If infections occur, they may require antibiotic therapy. Smoldering infections can also cause hyperglycemia or even ketoacidosis. To reduce the risk of infection, change the insertion site every 48 hours and secure well. Use warm water and soap, or a disinfectant skin wash, to cleanse the area. Skin reactions to the tape used to hold the needle in place may also occur. Paper-based or transparent plastic surgical tape reduces this risk.

If the pump malfunctions, ketoacidosis usually occurs much more rapidly than if a dose of injected insulin is missed. Pump programs usually depend on only rapidly disappearing regular insulin, while many injection programs include longer-acting insulin that maintains some hypoglycemic effect for a longer period of time.

The pump may fail to deliver insulin because of catheter obstruction or kinking, insulin aggregation or crystallization, or other mechanical malfunctions. The batteries can also wear out or become weak. When ill, you *must* follow aggressive sick-day rules because ketoacidosis can occur more rapidly.

With good pump performance and insulin flowing into your body constantly, improper adjustments—either poor dose decisions or mistakes setting the pump—can lead to insulin overdosage and severe hypoglycemia, clearly dangerous situations!

Since pumps carry more risks, they are not recommended for everyone. Pump users must be willing to test their blood frequently, pay close attention to the variable factors that affect diabetes control, such as diet and exercise, and have the judgment and willingness needed to play an active role in their own care.

Pump users should have a clear and realistic understanding of their goals. Many people think that the pump will prevent all complications or allow them to return to the carefree life of a nondiabetic person. Unfortunately, this seldom happens. Pump use provides no guarantees that complications will be avoided; it often requires more work than conventional or even MDI therapy.

Family support is important, too. It is preferable that pump users not live alone, both to provide this support and to reduce the risk in the event of serious hypoglycemia. Prescribing pump therapy is not for all physicians, either. It is important that physicians have experience with pump therapy and the support of diabetes educators to train pump users in proper self- care techniques.

## The benefits

On the positive side, pumps can be extremely effective in achieving normal or near-normal blood glucose levels in a person with type I diabetes. They are probably the most technologically advanced tool available for achieving this level of control (outside of a research laboratory) for those with unsatisfactory results from conventional treatment.

However, considering the risks involved, pump therapy frequently is considered when other methods of intensive insulin therapy are deemed inadequate. This decision may be based either on your past experience with MDI programs, or on the experienced opinion of your intensive insulin treatment team based on their assessments of your needs and goals.

The goal of this treatment is to achieve improved blood glucose control. In spite of the risks, this is the benefit, and for many, it is a tremendous benefit. If you determine that the risks of the suboptimal control that you have achieved using conventional therapy or MDI are greater than the risks and effort of pump therapy, then consider pump use. Be sure you conclude that pump use is likely to improve upon these other treatments.

If you are interested in using an insulin pump as part of your intensive insulin therapy, consult with your diabetes care team. Your diabetes care team may be the ones who first suggest using a pump. Regardless of who suggests it, the first step is discussion and a great deal of thought.

*Before* starting pump therapy, you must be thoroughly trained in its use, which may take several sessions with a diabetes educator who specializes in pump education. That educator should be up-to-date on the newest pump models and other equipment. It is beyond the scope of this manual to discuss models from which you may choose; our comments on pumps are general. See your health care team for specifics.

## General pump care

Routine maintenance is crucial, and many items need daily attention. Change batteries as recommended by the pump manufacturer and your health care team. Battery life may vary depending on pump use.

*Batteries*—Some pumps have self-contained batteries, and must be returned to the manufacturer when they wear out. Make sure you know the specific requirements of your pump's power source so you aren't left power-less!

*Syringes*—Pump syringe use is particularly important. Change the syringe daily, even if the syringe size allows more than one day's use. Daily changing of the syringe at a set time should be part of your routine; running over into the next day raises the chance that the syringe will run dry.

In preparing and using the syringe, it is very important to prevent air bubbles from entering the system; they take up space and can reduce the insulin delivered. One to two *inches* of air in the tubing take up a very significant volume and cause a drastic reduction in the amount of insulin that is delivered! Two inches of air equals, roughly, one unit of insulin. Air in the system can be a major problem in insulin pump therapy, and may actually result in ketoacidosis, especially when small doses of insulin are being used.

Since careful preparation of the syringe is so important, pump users should be instructed "one-on-one" prior to actually starting therapy. It is important to properly calculate the daily insulin volume, and be sure to include insulin that fills the tubing and needle. If you will be disconnecting and reconnecting the pump, be sure to prevent air from getting into the system, and maintain the proper insulin volume.

With all pumps, air bubbles can seep into the syringe or insulin from around the plunger. Drawing the plunger slowly rather than back and forth rapidly minimizes this leakage by preserving the silicon seal within the syringe.

It is sometimes helpful to overfill the insulin bottle with air so the syringe fills by itself rather than requiring the plunger to be pulled back manually. The catheter tubing should be pre-filled ("primed") by hand or by using the pump.

*The infusion set*—The catheter tubing, known as the "infusion set," can develop blockages, which can be a major cause of pump malfunction. Therefore, these sets should be routinely changed every other day. The tubing is usually 20 to 42 inches long, and the shorter the tubing, the less chance of occlusion. Most infusion-set tubing is 27-gauge and is attached to a 5/8-inch needle inserted subcutaneously.

*Skin care*—Some infusion sets have adhesive at the site of insertion to facilitate securing the tubing to the skin. Persons with sensitive skin and who are prone to rashes, dermatitis, or other skin problems are cautioned not to use these types of sets. Infusion sets without adhesive can be secured to the skin with transparent tapes (Op-site™ or Tegaderm™) which permit you to visually inspect the insertion site. Recurrent abscesses (skin infections—usually reddened, warm, raised areas, frequently oozing blood or yellowish fluid) may form at the insertion sites. If so, you may need to change the infusion sets daily. In general, washing the insertion sites with antiseptic wash (such as Hibiclens® or pHisoHex®) plus good general hygiene are essential. Nevertheless, when changing your infusion set, always look carefully for signs of infection.

The catheter needle should be bent at about a 45-degree angle before insertion (unless you are using one that requires straight-in insertion). This helps secure it in place and ensure that the insulin infuses subcutaneously (under the skin) rather than intradermally (into the skin). Once it is inserted, extra slack in the tubing should be looped a couple of times and taped down. Tubing should not be exposed to extreme heat or cold because extreme temperatures can affect the potency of the insulin.

Once the pump is running, attach it to the body in a comfortable and safe location. Many people attach it to a belt loop or the belt of a dress. Some patients sew pockets into clothing, and many men insert the pump into a shirt or coat pocket. Some women place their pumps in their bra, either on the side under the strap, or, if anatomy permits, in front. Velcro closures can be sewn into garments to allow the tubing to be run beneath them.

You may wish to come off of your pump for short periods of time for showers, swimming, and other activities. If you will be off the pump for longer than one hour, you will need to inject a dose of additional insulin. This time may vary slightly if exercise is involved, and your pump management team should give you guidelines. To come off the pump, leave the catheter needle inserted and disconnect the end of the catheter from the pump.

Cover the catheter hub and syringe tip with caps once they are disconnected.

To reconnect the pump, fill the hub of the tubing with insulin, either manually with a syringe or with the pump itself, to prevent bubble formation. (Be sure to consider this extra insulin volume that may be needed for reconnection when you're filling the pump and calculating the amounts of insulin you'll need.)

When manipulating the pump and tubing, use catheter clamps to prevent accidental bolusing of a dose of insulin. Also, do not hold the tubing up high, as the effect of gravity may draw insulin down and into the body as if a bolus of insulin were being delivered. Still, if problems persist with air getting into the system with this method of carefully disconnecting the tubing, the whole system may need to be removed, including removing the needle from your body.

*If you believe your pump is not working properly,* here are a few things to check before calling for help. First, disconnect the pump and program a bolus of 3 to 5 units. Watch for the insulin coming out of the infusion needle to be sure that a blockage has not developed in the needle or tubing. Insulin can occasionally aggregate (clump up) and cause such a blockage. When in doubt, change the infusion set.

Also be sure to check for leaks between the syringe and infusion set, the seal connecting the plastic tubing to the needle, or at the syringe-plunger site. Be sure there is no air in the tubing or large bubbles in the hub of the syringe or infusion set junction. Look at the needle insertion site for signs of inflammation or leakage, especially if the infusion set has not been changed recently. Keep your pump out of extreme heat or cold. Failure to do so can cause a malfunction, too. Finally, be sure that the batteries are good.

## Designing a pump program

The following are rough guidelines for designing a pump dosing program. **We do not recommend using this without guidance from a physician and a diabetes health care team.** We include it to indicate how you and the health care team will approach a pump program.

Designing a pump program is similar to designing a program using ultralente and regular: approximately half of the daily dose is the basal infusion, and the other half makes up the premeal bolus doses for glucose levels at or close to the normal range.

The total daily insulin dose is calculated at 0.5 units of insulin per kilogram of body weight. One half of this total is divided by 24, for the hourly basal infusion rate. The other half of the daily total is given as the premeal boluses, divided so that 40 percent is given as regular insulin before breakfast for a blood glucose in the normal range, and 30 percent each before lunch and supper. Regular doses are stepped up for incremental glucose levels above normal, and down for lower levels.

For example, assume that you weigh 167 lbs, or 76 kg. Your total daily insulin dose would be 76/2 or 38 units. Half of this is basal, or 19 units per day. Divided by 24 to determine hourly infusion rates, this is about 0.8 units per hour. Before breakfast, the regular insulin bolus for a glucose of about 100 to 149 mg/dl would be calculated as 0.4 x 19 = 7.6. You can start by either rounding up or down— down is more cautious! Try 7 units for a glucose in that range.

Prelunch and presupper doses would be calculated: 0.3 x 19 = 5.7. Try rounding up here to 6 units. Then, design the algorithm stepwise for higher and lower glucose values: Before breakfast, a glucose of 50 to 99 mg/dl would get 6 units, while a glucose of 150 to 199 mg/dl would get 8 units, and so on.

---

> **Again, do not design a pump program without
> guidance from your diabetes care team!**

Once this algorithm is designed, use the program and record glucose test results. Unless glucose levels are dangerously high or low, first address the fasting glucose levels, controlled primarily by the basal insulin dose. As long as overall glucose levels are generally high or low, adjust the single basal dose that runs for 24 hours. Adjust it in 0.1 to 0.2 unit increments usually.

However, if the daytime values differ from those overnight, and particularly fasting, you may need an alternate basal dose. For example, during the adjustment phase your target goal may be the low 100 mg/dl range. (Your ultimate goal once you get the hang of pump therapy will be arrived at by you and your health care team.) If, with adjustments, the glucose values during the day begin to approach the low 100 mg/dl range while the fasting values are still too high, consider an alternate basal dose during the latter part of the night. Alternate basal doses are discussed later in this chapter.

When fasting glucose levels are at or close to the target range and the values are too high later in the day, begin adjusting the regular insulin dose scales. The general rules for adjustments of intensive insulin therapies discussed earlier apply to pump users as well.

The basal rate and the algorithm outlining bolus doses generally should *not* be changed at the same time, because it becomes difficult to sort out the effect of each change. However, under supervision of the pump care team, multiple dose adjustment allows more rapid achievement of desired goals.

It's important for every pump user to talk with his or her management team about how to adjust pump basal rates and algorithms.

Frequently, close communication is needed between the patient and the health care team, so it is recommended that persons using a pump live not more than a two-hour drive from the team unless special arrangements have been made.

## Pumps and sick days

The usual sick day rules for insulin dose adjustments, with certain modifications, apply to pump users too. The usual recommendation at the Joslin Diabetes Center is to increase the basal infusion rate(s) by 50 percent on clearly defined sick days. The boluses are then increased too, using a quantity of insulin that has been predetermined in discussions with the pump care team.

Often, pump boluses are increased by an amount equal to 10 to 20 percent of the sum of the *total* daily insulin doses. (**NOTE:** This means basal *plus* boluses, calculated for a normal range glucose value!) Extra boluses may also be needed.

You should calculate your "sick day incremental dose" as follows: Ten percent of the total daily dose is used on sick days for blood glucose values between 240 mg/dl and 400 mg/dl without ketones. Twenty percent is used for values over 400 mg/dl, or levels between 240 mg/dl and 400 mg/dl if ketones are present.

When ill, you should check your blood glucose level every four hours around the clock. A reading over 240 mg/dl qualifies for extra insulin, as a bolus of the appropriate amount of your sick day incremental dose. If it is time for a routine dose of insulin (such as before a meal) add this incremental dose to the usual insulin bolus quantity and give it before the meal.

With use of an algorithm during sick days, the bolus doses will already be higher before you add the catch-up. The nature of your algorithm—the amount of insulin given and the size of the routine dose increases for higher glucose levels—will determine how to approach the sick-day increases.

Input from your pump care team is essential *before* you get sick, so you will know what to do in advance. Discuss what constitutes a sick day. Be sure that you understand how you should use these *general* guidelines when *you* get sick.

Remember, sick days require more insulin. Be sure to check the insulin supply in the syringe frequently!

After you increase both the basal and the boluses, if your blood glucose level does not come into an acceptable range within 2 to 3 hours, remove the pump and use injected insulin, with the alternative split-mix dose, plus standard sick-day rules.

Sick days are not times to troubleshoot, and if there is any question of whether the pump is functioning properly, use insulin injections instead. Any suggestions of ketoacidosis—frequent urination, high sugar levels, ketones in the urine—should prompt an immediate switch to injected insulin plus a trip to the physician or emergency room, because ketoacidosis can come on quite rapidly.

Never hesitate to temporarily come off of the pump and use injected insulin in any time of trouble or confusion. Many physicians who do not specialize in the care of diabetes may still be quite capable of properly treating an emergency, but may have absolutely *no idea* how to use a pump!

Clearly, in case of an emergency, choose the best qualified physician or hospital available. But if you still have any doubt about the management of your diabetes with the pump, disconnect it and use injected insulin until you can get in touch with someone knowledgeable who can help you. In a pinch, pump companies often have patient representatives you can reach by phone who may be helpful.

Insulin therapy is best individualized, and this is never so true as with pump therapy in general, and pump therapy on sick days, especially. The above guidelines are for general information. All patients using pump therapy must be quite clear on their specific sick day instructions *before* they become ill.

## Exercise adjustments

Adjustments for exercise vary widely from person to person, and trial and error is the best way to determine appropriate adjustments for a given amount of exercise. Pump users are no exception. There are many ways to adjust for exercise: you can reduce the basal infusion rate during exercise, you can take the pump off if the exercise is strenuous, or you can eat additional food.

In general, pumps should not be worn during contact or water sports. However, pump manufacturers are making innovations in their pumps that may lead to waterproof, shockproof equipment. For sexual activity, the pump can be removed or worn, depending on personal preference. Most chose to remove it.

Each pump user should develop his or her approach to exercise adjustments, but general guidelines can help. See Chapter 8 for discussion of exercise and intensive insulin therapy. For those using a pump, exercise poses specific concerns.

If the exercise occurs up to three hours from the last insulin bolus, hypoglycemia can occur. Additional food is helpful to prevent hypoglycemia, but if the activity is anticipated, giving about 50 percent of the usual premeal bolus is an alternative. For prolonged, less strenuous exercise, such as two to three hours of bicycling or walking, reducing the basal rate by 30 to 50 percent may be preferable.

In general, consult pump management teams for guidance about adjustments and manipulations to accommodate exercise. And keep careful records, so you can later review what alterations were made, how long and how strenuous the activity was, and the effect on your blood glucose levels. Then you can learn what works for *you*.

### Pump vacations

Pump vacations are times when a regular user does not use his or her pump. These may occur due to equipment malfunction, other illness, travel, catheter insertion site infection or inflammation, or just simply periods of time for a break from the intensive self-management that pump treatment requires.

Pump vacations are usually longer than the short-term pump disconnections for showers, exercise, or sexual activity and usually are measured in terms of days off of pump therapy rather than minutes or hours.

It is essential to have calculated an alternate insulin dose to give by syringe injection. It is always good to anticipate a possible emergency pump vacation due to equipment malfunction and have this alternative insulin dose ready. Determine the exact alternative treatment doses with the help of your pump care team.

If you need a dose immediately and you cannot reach your pump team, some general guidelines help. Calculate the quantity of insulin given as the pump basal over a 24-hour period and give that amount as two injections of NPH or lente insulin. Usually, two-thirds of this total is given before breakfast, and one-third before supper. This same pump algorithm for regular premeal insulin boluses can be used for injected regular insulin at those same times.

Remember, however, the prelunch regular insulin will peak at about the same time as the morning NPH or lente, so you may need to alter either of these doses. You may consider taking the second injection of NPH or lente at bedtime so it peaks at the end of your sleep period. Further dose adjustments may be necessary if the vacation is to be prolonged, if activity is different, or if the vacation is due to an illness or injury.

Anyone using a pump may encounter the need for an emergency pump vacation, but *elective* vacations may not be advisable for everyone. People who might have a dangerous deterioration in their control should avoid them.

In general, if you are feeling tired, frustrated, or "burned out" with pump therapy, start by talking with your health care team. Discuss your options before abandoning the pump on your own.

## Summary

Pump use is not for everyone; indeed, it is really for a select few. It is a major undertaking that requires understanding, patience, and perseverance. However, it can very effectively approach normal insulin action and glucose metabolism for someone with type I diabetes. When the hard work, attention, and persistence pay off and this treatment proves successful, the rewards of improved diabetes control and a more flexible lifestyle are often worth the effort.

# Chapter Eight

# Exercise and the Intensive Plan

## What's this section about?

- Why does exercise help control?

- How do you plan an exercise program?

- When do you need to adjust diabetes treatment to exercise?

- Is food a factor?

We hear much these days about the virtues of exercise. Those of us in the medical profession encourage our patients to exercise, and you can hardly walk through a shopping center today without seeing window displays for sporting goods, exercise clothes, vacations to exercise resorts, or some other product related to fitness. Exercise is definitely "in!"

And for people with diabetes, exercise is especially important. Along with insulin and the meal plan, it is one of the three primary factors that influence glucose metabolism. In fact, exercise probably was one of the earliest forms of diabetes treatment, although it was not always recognized as such.

## Why exercise helps

Exercise should be fun as well as good for you. For people with diabetes, it has not been shown conclusively that exercise directly prevents diabetic complications. However, we do know that in persons without diabetes, exercise reduces the risk of vascular problems such as heart disease and peripheral vascular disease (hardening of the arteries).

Sustained aerobic exercise reduces the levels of blood lipids (fats, such as cholesterol) as well as lowering blood pressure. It promotes good blood circulation and strengthens the heart. It is reasonable to assume that a person with diabetes will enjoy the same cardiovascular benefits, but exercise also has special importance in blood glucose metabolism. It both lowers blood glucose levels, and increases insulin sensitivity, so the insulin works more effectively.

Finally, do not overlook the psychological benefits of exercise as an excellent way to manage stress and work out frustrations. Many people feel better after exercise, are less anxious, and can cope better with life's little problems. Exercise can also improve your self-image as you become more physically fit.

## Exercise without diabetes

Muscle normally uses glucose and free fatty acids (fat) as fuel to provide needed energy. The glucose comes either directly from the blood or from glucagon stored in liver or muscle tissue. Initially, short bursts of activity are fueled by glucose from either the blood or glycogen from muscle. However, after about 15 minutes of activity, the glucose source is the liver, often provided by conversion from amino acids (the building blocks of protein, particularly one called alanine). After about 30 minutes of exercise, the body begins to get more of its energy from the free fatty acids.

After exercise, many of the glycogen stores in the liver and muscle have been depleted, and the body begins rebuilding them. This usually takes 4 to 6 hours but can take up to 12 or even 24 hours if the exertion has been intense. Insulin is needed for this replenishment, but there also must be enough glucose in the blood from which to make the glycogen.

In people with diabetes, if the blood glucose levels are too low after exercise, the rebuilding of the glycogen stores can result in hypoglycemic reactions over the next few hours ("lag" effect) as blood glucose is used up by this process.

## Exercise with diabetes

For people with diabetes, the ability to maintain proper glucose/energy balance is determined by how well their diabetes is controlled, how much insulin they presently have available, and their level of hydration. Theoretically, someone with well-controlled diabetes and the proper insulin/glucose balance can handle exercise as well as someone who does not have diabetes.

With less than optimal control, however, the ability to handle the metabolic needs of exercise is reduced. With "fair" diabetes control, glycogen stores are often diminished. Thus, the available fuels (glucose) run out sooner and the body starts to burn the free fatty acids for fuel, producing ketones.

Very poor control further worsens the problem of getting proper fuels. The overabundance of glucose in the blood is unavailable as an energy source because of the lack of insulin. Reduced levels of insulin also permit the liver to make more glucose. It is as if the body tissues, starved for sugar, think that more is needed and they produce more and more. This becomes even worse as glucose production continues to be stimulated by the increasing energy demand of the exercising muscles.

Unable to use glucose, the body turns to its alternative fuel, free fatty acids. (Remember, insufficient insulin allows the free fatty acids back into the circulation for use as an alternative fuel.) When fat is metabolized, ketones are produced. Thus, in a person with poorly controlled diabetes who is exercising, glucose levels keep rising, and ketones are produced as free fatty acids are metabolized as an alternative fuel source. Obviously, this metabolic picture is not optimal for good physical performance—or good health, for that matter!

For those in good control, exercise should not cause these difficulties, and in fact, has many benefits. As long as the diabetes control is good and *the proper amount of insulin is present,* increased activity uses additional glucose without any increased insulin need. Since working muscle is more sensitive to insulin action than muscle at rest, it uses more glucose for fuel per unit of insulin than does resting muscle. Thus, activity is one of the three major factors affecting blood glucose levels, along with food and insulin.

Exercise can reduce blood glucose levels in the short term. And regular exercise increases insulin sensitivity in persons with diabetes, helping available insulin work more efficiently.

## The exercise program

*Types of exercise*—Endurance training is exercise that uses a great deal of energy, stimulating the heart and lungs, and uses most of the body muscles for at least 15 to 20 minutes each session. Strength training, such as weight lifting, applies heavy resistance to specific muscle groups. Most physicians and exercise physiologists recommend endurance exercise as the most useful activity for adults because of the beneficial stress effect on the cardiovascular and metabolic systems. The training most recommended for people with diabetes is listed here.

### Physical activities for people with diabetes

**Individual activities:**

| | |
|---|---|
| Brisk walking | Running or jogging |
| Swimming | Bicycling (including stationary) |
| Dancing | Skipping rope |
| Rowing | Skiing (downhill and cross-country) |
| Badminton | Skating (ice and roller) |
| Wrestling | Golf (with brisk walking only!) |
| Fencing | Stair climbing |
| Calisthenics | Tennis |
| Handball | Squash |
| Racquetball | |

**Team activities:**

| | |
|---|---|
| Soccer | Volleyball (vigorous only!) |
| Basketball | Hockey (ice and field) |
| Lacrosse | |

**Other activities, if done at the proper intensity:**

| | |
|---|---|
| Digging | Wood cutting and splitting |
| Lawn mowing | Farming |

## Evaluation before starting

Anyone starting an exercise program should first be evaluated by a physician. This is important at *any* age. While older individuals may be concerned with heart, lung, or circulatory damage, many young people with long-term diabetes unfortunately still have a potential for similar problems. Better safe than sorry! Your physician will determine the extent of your pre-exercise evaluation, but consultation is essential.

Many people reading an intensive diabetes manual such as this one have diabetes in excellent control. If you have any doubts, however, check with your health care team. Any complications must be monitored during the exercise program. Persons with retinopathy (diabetic eye disease), for example, should discuss exercise with their ophthalmologist.

Some exercise can increase blood pressure, which may cause retinal hemorrhages in people with retinopathy, or further damage kidneys that diabetes has already affected. Your feet should also be carefully checked.

## Prescribing exercise

Good exercise programs have four characteristics: (1) the type of activity, (2) the intensity, (3) the duration of each session, and (4) the frequency of the sessions. Consider each of these in planning an exercise program.

It is beyond the scope of this manual to detail the actual design and function of an exercise program. However, for a properly designed exercise program, speak to your physician and get help from an exercise physiologist, who should be available as part of your diabetes care team.

## Adjusting diabetes treatment to exercise

For people with diabetes, exercise does lower the blood glucose levels. This is very beneficial, but you must make compensatory adjustments in the two other major factors controlling blood glucose levels—food and insulin—so your diabetes control remains in proper balance.

Remember, too, that all exercise is not part of a formal exercise or recreation program. An active day of shopping, additional work around the house or on the job, or even sexual activity, may have the same effect on diabetes as an exercise session and should be approached accordingly.

The first rule of exercise and diabetes is that *no* exercise should be performed if the diabetes is out of control: that is, if you have a blood glucose level over 300 mg/dl, especially if urine ketones are present. These findings suggest an insulin lack, which can cause an increased blood glucose level or a worsening of the ketosis with exercise.

To maintain proper diabetes control during and after an exercise session, you must adjust food and insulin doses. Ultimately, the best way to determine how much is to keep careful records of blood glucose levels, insulin dose, food adjustments, and some idea of the amount of activity you are involved in.

Then study your records and from your own experiences, determine the best adjustments for each activity. Blood testing before and after exercise is a minimum; it is also important to test blood *during* an exercise session and a few hours afterwards, looking for low blood glucose levels.

## Insulin and exercise

It is often a challenge to have just the right amount of insulin present both during and after exercise. There are a number of ways that exercise can affect insulin's action.

Injected insulin acts over a prolonged period of time because its chemical properties have been altered to prolong absorption. During exercise, this injected insulin is being absorbed continuously—you cannot turn it off. Therefore, you must carefully assess the residual effects of insulin previously injected.

Theoretically, this is less of a problem for those using pumps, as continuous subcutaneous infusions produce less of a reservoir of injected insulin that must be absorbed, and the insulin effect can be altered more accurately when a change is needed. However, even with pumps, if you exercise shortly after an insulin bolus, this problem may still be present.

Paradoxically, exercise sometimes frees insulin that has been inactivated because it is bound up and sequestered in various "corners of the body." This actually increases the available insulin during exercise!

Certain intensive diabetes programs are more easily adapted to exercise than others. Daytime regular doses used with overnight intermediate insulin, for example, can be adjusted to produce desired dips in the insulin levels. These dips occur reliably because there is no other insulin—no basal—acting over this time period. The only insulin acting is the regular insulin, which you can reduce to produce a lower blood insulin level.

However, reducing the regular insulin in a program that uses ultralente to produce a basal effect may not lead to a low enough insulin level to prevent hypoglycemia. Reliance on a combination of the regular with the longer acting and less predictable ultralente also may not allow precise enough control at the time of the exercise.

People using intensive diabetes programs are frequently frustrated when they discover that their glucose levels are higher after exercise than they were before. Their first thought is that they had an unrecognized reaction during exercise, and they perform multiple blood glucose tests before, during, and after exercise looking for evidence of hypoglycemia. Often, they can find no sign of a reaction. Was their pre-exercise glucose value too high? Probably not, since they most likely checked and it was not over 300 mg/dl and no ketones were present. Correctly, they assumed that, with these findings, it was all right to exercise.

So, what happened?

Certainly, hypoglycemia could still be an explanation. Also, if the pre-exercise glucose was too high, clearly there was not enough insulin present at the start of exercise. With insufficient insulin, exercise would cause the glucose level to rise and ketones to be produced as the body uses fat as an alternative fuel. But could there have been insufficient insulin present with a pre-exercise blood glucose level *below* 300 mg/dl?

Yes! The insulin level at the start of the exercise could have been dropping! In this circumstance, there would have been enough insulin left from the previous injection to hold the pre-exercise glucose level in a good range. But because the action of that insulin dose was waning and, with the passage of time spent exercising, the insulin level dropped further, finally it reached a point where there *was* insufficient insulin.

With too little insulin, the liver produces more glucose than is needed, fat is burned for energy-producing ketones, and the whole "exercise with insulin lack" scenario takes place in spite of a sufficient amount of insulin at the beginning of exercise. In addition, adrenalin secretion is often increased during exercise, and adrenalin causes a further rise in blood glucose levels.

The solution? Adjust the insulin doses so more insulin is acting during the exercise period. Often a longer acting insulin such as NPH, lente, or ultralente is increased, although regular insulin can be used. Obviously, there is a fine line between too much insulin and too little, but sometimes when more insulin is needed, additional food must also be consumed for proper glucose levels.

This problem typically arises first thing in the morning, a popular time for exercising. The intermediate or long-acting insulin from the night before is wearing off, and the morning insulin has not yet started working. In fact, people often postpone their insulin until after their exercise, finding that if they take regular insulin before, they become hypoglycemic during the morning. However, postbreakfast blood glucose levels are frequently quite high.

This problem is frequently solved by increasing the previous night's insulin dose. At times, compensatory decreases in the presupper regular insulin or increases in the bedtime snack, or both, are needed. Occasionally, if this does not work, some people take a small injection of regular insulin before exercising (plus a small snack), then exercise, then take their normal morning injection (minus a few units to make up for the regular taken earlier), then have breakfast. It is a bit cumbersome, but for those with high goals, it can work nicely.

Clearly, the timing of exercise can influence blood glucose levels. For example, late afternoon exercise would coincide with the peak time of the morning NPH or lente insulin rather than at a low point, as in the previous example. A reduction of the dose might be needed—either the prelunch regular or the morning intermediate or long-acting insulin. Trial and error often will tell you which dose to adjust.

Always consider how the timing of exercise relates to insulin action, especially when trying to figure out why exercise days may differ. Ideally, the best time for exercise sessions is at least an hour after a meal—and ideally after the largest meal of the day, dinner. In addition, if you can do your major daily workout at the same time every day, you will become adept at the adjustments needed.

## Regular physical activity

People who participate regularly in vigorous physical activity experience metabolic adaptations so that each exercise session does not affect blood glucose levels as much as you might expect. People without diabetes who exercise regularly have lower basal insulin levels and require less insulin at mealtime, probably because they have more insulin receptors, their insulin works more efficiently, and fewer catecholamines (adrenalin and related substances) are secreted for a given amount of activity.

For people with type I diabetes, as conditioning improves, insulin requirements often change (usually diminishing), and insulin and food adjustments to compensate for activity variations may decrease. Some people also experience less of a lag effect as well.

## Planned and unplanned exercise

Many people cover activity successfully by adjusting food as well as insulin. In fact, while you may have to reduce the insulin dose when starting an exercise program, once the activity becomes routine, you will know how much you need to adjust your insulin to accommodate planned exercise. By planning when you exercise, eating extra food to cover your insulin won't usually be necessary. You will adjust your insulin to accommodate planned exercise. You can use snack adjustment to accommodate for unplanned exercise. The need for a snack in response to unplanned exercise is affected by the quantity of insulin acting during and after the exercise, the time since the last meal, and the duration and intensity of the planned exercise.

Part of planning your exercise means scheduling it for one to two hours after you eat—not two or more hours after a meal, when you won't have enough food on board to cover the exercise. If you exercise more than two hours after a meal, even this "planned" exercise may require a snack. Unplanned activity often requires snacks, but the risk of hypoglycemia will still be high, even if you snack. Snacking recommendations for unplanned exercise are summarized and some possible snack foods are listed in the tables that follow. Remember, the time of day affects the amounts of snacks needed, so keep good records and learn from your experience! Also, no matter how confident you are, always have some quick carbohydrate handy, just in case.

Some people find that even when planning their exercise their pre-exercise insulin adjustments aren't enough to prevent hypoglycemia hours after their exercise as a result of the lag effect. If you fall into this category, you may also want to adjust your insulin dose following exercise. For people on intensive therapy with normal post-exercise blood glucose levels, this may be extremely important.

In the case of all-day planned activities, you will find that you need to both adjust your insulin and eat extra snacks to prevent low blood sugars. The snacking adjustments for unplanned exercise on page 135 will work for you in this situation, used together with the insulin adjustments for planned exercise on page 133. This practice is most important for day-long activities like cross-country skiing or hiking. The insulin adjustment scenario on page 137 will help you understand how to do this.

### Fluids

Fluids are important too; dehydration can worsen diabetes control. Much fluid is lost through sweating, so be sure to drink enough before starting exercise. Water is best because it is most easily absorbed. You may also need fluids during exercise, especially for activity that causes profuse sweating, such as prolonged exercise or a workout in warm weather.

## Weight loss

With weight loss as a goal, you should place your greatest emphasis on insulin dose reductions rather than snacking. This requires careful planning, because insulin dose adjustments must often be made well before the activity. Look for patterns of blood glucose levels following exercise and make adjustments in your insulin to take these into account. The insulin adjustment scenario described on page 137 will help you understand how to do this.

| Insulin adjustment guidelines for exercise | | |
|---|---|---|
| Adjust the insulin **acting** during exercise using these guidelines | | |
| ·Percent to decrease peaking insulin | Intensity of exercise | Duration of exercise |
| 0% | Low, moderate or high intensity | Short duration |
| 5% | Low intensity | Intermediate to long |
| 10% | Moderate | Intermediate |
| 20% | Moderate | Long |
| 20% | High | Intermediate |
| 30 to 50% | High | Long |

**Duration of exercise:** short = less than 30 minutes (not necessary to adjust insulin); intermediate = 30 to 60 minutes; long = 60 minutes or more.

**Intensity of duration:** high intensity = high end of target heart rate; moderate intensity = low end of target heart rate; low intensity = not in target zone.

| Snacking for unplanned exercise | | | |
|---|---|---|---|
| **Type of exercise and examples** | **If blood glucose is:** | **Additional carbohydrate and/or protein** | **Food suggested** |
| Short duration (less than 30 minutes) and of *low* to moderate intensity | Under 100 mg/dl | 10 to 15 grams carbohydrate | 1 bread or 1 fruit |
| | 100 mg/dl to 240 mg/dl | May not be necessary to increase food | |
| **Examples:** Walking a mile, leisurely bicycling for less than 30 minutes | | | |
| Intermediate duration (about 1 hour) and of moderate intensity | Under 100 mg/dl | 30 grams carbohydrate + 7 or 8 grams protein | 1 fruit + 1 bread + 1 meat |
| | 100 mg/dl to 180 mg/dl | 15 grams of carbohydrate + 7 or 8 grams protein | 1 bread + 1 meat |
| | 180 mg/dl to 240 mg/dl | 10 to 15 grams of carbohydrate (food may not be necessary) | 1 bread or 1 fruit |
| **Examples:** Tennis, swimming, jogging leisurely, bicycling, gardening, golfing, low-impact beginners' aerobic class | | | |
| Long duration (over 1 hour) and of moderate intensity | Same as for intermediate duration but add 1 fruit or 1 bread for each hour after the initial hour | | |

| Snacking for unplanned exercise (cont.) | | | |
|---|---|---|---|
| **Type of exercise and examples** | **If blood glucose is:** | **Additional carbohydrate and/or protein** | **Food suggested** |
| Intermediate duration (about 1 hour) and of high intensity | Less than 100 mg/dl | 30 to 50 grams carbohydrate + 14 to 15 grams protein* | 2 breads+ 2 meats + 1 milk |
| | 100 mg/dl to 180 mg/dl | 15 grams of carbohydrate + 7 or 8 grams protein | 1 bread + 1 meat |
| | 180 mg/dl to 240 mg/dl | 15 grams of carbohydrate | 1 bread or 1 fruit |
| **Examples:** Racquetball, high-intensity aerobics, strenuous swimming or cycling, and running | | | |
| Long duration (over 1 hour) and of high intensity | Same as for intermediate duration but add 2 breads or 2 fruits for each hour after the initial hour* | | |

* Add 1 fruit or 1 bread for each hour after the first 2 hours.

## Snack foods for exercise

### Foods containing 10 to 15 grams of carbohydrate

Small piece of fresh fruit
2 tablespoons of raisins
5 to 7 dried apricot halves
4 to 6 crackers
1 slice of bread

### Foods containing 7 to 8 grams of protein

1 ounce of low-fat cheese
1/4 cup of low-fat cottage cheese
1 ounce of poultry or lean meat
1/4 cup of tuna or salmon
1 tablespoon peanut butter

## Summary

Sometimes, people on intensive insulin therapy feel frustrated because exercise seems to confuse their efforts. It can be more difficult to quantitate, anticipate, and therefore compensate for the variations in eating. Occasionally people quit their exercise programs in despair. DON'T! Exercise IS worth the effort. In the long run, regular exercise will help improve your glucose control and overall health.

## Planned insulin adjustments for exercise

Premeal boluses of insulin may be substantially reduced or even eliminated before or after exercise. Adjust the insulin having the most effect during the exercise period. If this insulin is regular insulin, reduce the algorithm scale by 1 to 2 units for a specific glucose range. Blood glucose values should be taken immediately after exercise. If the blood glucose is 100 mg/dl or less, this indicates that the circulating insulin is still too high. If this is the case, reduce the algorithm by an additional unit for the next exercise session.

The algorithm scale associated with the next injection of regular insulin may also need to be reduced. This should be done if the exercise is ending within one to two hours of the next injection. This will help control any lag effect you may experience.

When an algorithm is not being used, the same principle of reducing the insulin acting during the activity still applies. Start by decreasing the dosage of insulin acting during the exercise by 10 percent of the total insulin dose for the day. You may also need to reduce the post-exercise dose to compensate for the lag effect.

To determine the percentage of insulin to reduce, correlate the planned exercise intensity and duration on the chart on page 133. For intensive programs, this would apply to the regular insulin dose. Intermediate insulin, if peaking during or after the activity, may also be adjusted. However, ultralente should not be reduced for routine exercise and is only adjusted for activities occurring over several days, such as long-distance cycling. Similarly, reduction of the post-exercise insulin dose may be needed to compensate for the lag effect.

Blood glucose testing is the only way to evaluate the effectiveness of insulin adjustments. If a hypoglycemic reaction occurs during or after exercise, decrease the insulin dose even more the next time the same exercise is done. Keep records of test results and adjustments. Insulin adjustments can be used only when exercise is planned.

# Chapter Nine

# Pregnancy and Intensive Diabetes Therapy

## What's this section about?

- Why is good physiologic control so important during pregnancy?

- How does intensive diabetes therapy work for pregnant women?

Efforts to achieve excellent diabetes control have significantly improved the chances for women with diabetes to have successful pregnancies and healthy babies. At one time, pregnancy for women with diabetes was a major threat to both mother and child, but today the maternal death rate is as low as for the general population, and the infant mortality is significantly improved over what it was.

Today, the focus is close monitoring of both the diabetes and the developing fetus. Details of the approach to pregnancy in women with diabetes can be found in other Joslin and American Diabetes Association publications.

Since good diabetes control is important in a successful pregnancy, many women choose intensive insulin therapy to achieve it.

## Why good control is especially important during pregnancy

While most diabetes care professionals believe that the best blood glucose control is in everyone's best interest, some of the strongest evidence applies to pregnant women.

There is evidence that achieving good physiologic ("tight") control before and during pregnancy reduces the chances that the fetus will be born with significant malformations. Major organs of the body are formed in the first trimester (the first three months) of pregnancy, when good control is especially important. Severe malformations may lead to fetal death, and miscarriage is more common in women with poorly controlled diabetes.

Since some pregnancies are unplanned, a woman may be well into her first trimester before knowing she is pregnant. If she has diabetes and has not been paying special attention, she may have gone through much of this critical period with dangerously poor control. Therefore, improved control *before* conception is the ideal goal, and this usually means planning your pregnancy.

Finally, good control helps the mother through her pregnancy with a minimum of difficulty and discomfort. The added stress of a pregnancy to a body already affected by diabetes can be minimized if glucose metabolism is as good as it can be.

A woman with diabetes is more likely to have a successful pregnancy if she maintains the best possible control for at least three months before conception. Your health care team should work with you to determine how good your control should be.

Clearly, some women may already have achieved this level of diabetes control before pregnancy is even contemplated, but for those who have not, this is an important part of caring for your as-yet unborn and even as-yet unconceived child.

To achieve better control, many women see their physician more frequently and work more intensively at controlling the variables that affect diabetes. Changes in your body during the nine month gestational period may affect your blood glucose metabolism. Most women find that they need less insulin during the first trimester, but insulin requirements begin to rise during the second trimester to a maximum during the third. Therefore, close attention to blood monitoring and glycohemoglobin tests are important.

### Do you need intensive insulin therapy?

Not everyone anticipating a pregnancy will need intensive diabetes therapy as outlined in this book to achieve the necessary level of diabetes control to have a healthy baby. However, most women will need to manage their diabetes more intensively using one of the methods described in this book! All women in the DCCT study who became pregnant were put on some form of intensive therapy.

Most women who enter a pregnancy with noninsulin dependent diabetes mellitus (type II diabetes) or who develop diabetes during pregnancy (gestational diabetes) must pay close attention to the variables but do not need formal intensive therapy with its adjustable insulin doses. Fixed doses, perhaps adjusted to accommodate for activity or eating variations, often are sufficient if these variations are held to a minimum.

In general, the woman who will need intensive diabetes therapy to prepare for a pregnancy is likely to be the woman who will need intensive therapy to achieve good to excellent control when *not* pregnant. She may not have chosen the rigors of intensive therapy before pregnancy became an issue, feeling her control was satisfactory. But with pregnancy, her goals may be higher.

Pregnancy is a marvelous motivator! Women know that top-notch control is important, and the intensity of the effort is for a finite period, so they often are willing to put much more effort into their control—even intensified conventional control—during pregnancy.

As a result of the increased motivation and the increased attention by the health care team, improvements usually take place even before significant changes in treatment are made. For many, the frequent contact with the health care team for program adjustments may be sufficient.

Therefore, prepregnant and pregnant women undertake intensive therapy for the same reason anyone else would: high goals for diabetes control. The challenge of self-management is the same whether a woman is pregnant or not, so it is important that the woman attempting intensive therapy during pregnancy meet the same qualifications discussed in earlier chapters. The alternatives—intensifying the conventional approach and more frequent health team visits—can often achieve satisfactory improvements in control for those who do not meet those qualifications.

Intensive diabetes therapy for women who are pregnant or plan to be is not appreciably different from that for anyone else. Of course, other issues must be attended to, such as proper nutrition for both you and your developing fetus, and proper obstetrical care. However, the approach to insulin dose adjustment and testing is the same.

Since intensive therapy is undertaken because of high goals, gauge your success in terms of self glucose test results and the glycohemoglobin. To lower the latter as much as possible, frequent monitoring of postmeal and middle-of-the-night blood glucose levels is essential. The closer these are to targeted levels, the lower the resulting glycohemoglobin is likely to be.

While we have stressed that intensive diabetes therapy must be managed by a physician or health care team familiar with this approach to diabetes care, clearly this is even more important when you are pregnant. And if your diabetes health care team is not already affiliated with an obstetrician or obstetrical group familiar with the management of women with diabetes, find one. Then, make sure those managing your diabetes and those managing your pregnancy keep in touch!

## Summary

With proper care, your chances of having a healthy baby are greatly increased today, compared with times past. That care should start with education. Learn about what the combination of diabetes and pregnancy means to you and to your child so you can be an active member of your health care team and make informed choices.

# Chapter Ten

# Psychological Concerns

■ Is your mental outlook important for intensive diabetes management?

■ Who are the best patients?

■ How can you prepare yourself mentally for this program?

Early in a physician's or nurse's training, we learn that to consider only a patient's physical ailments is to do only half the job. Any medical condition, from a simple cold to a terminal illness, is accompanied by the person's psychological response to the condition. These responses differ, depending on individual personality differences, as well as the severity of the condition, the actual or anticipated duration, and the treatments that are required. But individual responses always must be considered. They frequently play an important role in the recommended treatment.

Diabetes treatment must also address a person's psychological response to this condition, particularly if the treatment is intensive diabetes therapy. Health care providers and their patients must never lose sight of an individual's psychological state as he or she is considering, initiating, and managing this treatment. Together, we must explore the issues that have affected a patient's choices. Once therapy has started, we and our patients must not only assess the response of blood glucose levels, we must also gauge our patient's personal responses to treatment. As people live with intensive therapy, we, their health care providers, and they must talk together frequently to identify signs of perfectionism, frustration, "burn-out" or poor judgment.

## Psychological responses to diabetes

No one with diabetes can live a life quite as free as someone without it. Complete freedom to eat, to do as you please when you please, to be as active as you want whenever you want, is not feasible. Freedom is often tethered to insulin action patterns, test results, and eating schedules, which can result in depression, anger, or despair.

Yet, in some people, the emotions stirred by the challenge of mastering this condition also create a sense of accomplishment at conquering its complexities. Many are also encouraged by the hope that good self-care and advances in research will give them a better life than people with diabetes of generations past.

We health care providers try to foster these more positive emotions, by encouraging interest and self-management by people with diabetes, and involvement and support by others close to them. We try to show people that diabetes does not mean sacrificing life's many pleasures, just that they must work harder to achieve them.

Written on the west stairwell wall in the older section of the Joslin Diabetes Center is a quote from Isadore, Archbishop of Seville, who lived from 570 to 636 A.D: "Learn as if you were to live forever. Live as if you would die tomorrow."

With diabetes, be optimistic that your life will be long, and work to make it full of good health through effort and study. Yet, value each day and live it to its fullest. Balance what is needed for your good health with what it takes to live a life of quality. Sometimes it may seem that the efforts to achieve good health are overwhelming, but remember the reasons these efforts are important.

### Coping mechanisms

Many people approach diabetes as they would any undesirable situation—by denying it has happened. Denial occurs when you subconsciously behave as if the unpleasant situation does not really exist. If this leads to ignoring self-care, it is harmful. However, if it does not affect self-care, it may enable you to maintain a positive attitude despite adversity. Another word for this response is "optimism," and it can be a good approach as long as you maintain proper self-care.

Some people respond to diabetes with *fear*—fear of reactions, fear of complications, fear of early death. Memories of trouble experienced by others with diabetes may stimulate fear. Fear and anxiety are poor motivators. Sometimes when people fear diabetes, they "freeze" and cannot handle even the most basic self-care. Others become so driven to perfection, hoping to prevent the feared outcome, that they develop unrealistic expectations for their treatment. Still others become so driven by their fear that they make improper decisions. These responses make for a miserable existence. *Guilt* may also be a response to diabetes. Guilt that, by having diabetes and potentially becoming ill or disabled, you are letting others down, shirking responsibilities to family, friends, and employers. When this occurs, glucose levels that are too high or too low become "bad test results" and the failure to achieve desired goals becomes a reflection of personal worth.

## How long will I live?

This question plagues many people, but it is particularly poignant for people with diabetes. We cannot answer this question, nor can we say for sure what will lengthen your life. A better question, perhaps, is "How well will I live?"

While we cannot predict longevity or which complications will arise, predicting the quality of life may be more within our grasp. For those with diabetes, quality of life can be affected by how well you control your sugars and how you integrate self-care efforts into your lifestyle.

Achieving success in controlling diabetes while integrating that control program comfortably into your lifestyle are two reasons that you might consider intensive insulin therapy.

## Psychological aspects of choosing intensive diabetes therapy

Earlier, we indicated three reasons for undertaking intensive diabetes therapy:

1. Desire to achieve normal blood glucose patterns.

2. Failure to achieve even minimally acceptable levels of control with standard therapy, in spite of great personal effort.

3. Variable lifestyle or schedules that are incompatible with less flexible conventional treatments.

It is sometimes helpful to question further the "reasons behind these reasons":

- Why do you want to achieve normal blood glucose levels?

- Why are you unhappy with your present level of diabetes control?

- How do you balance variations in your lifestyle with your diabetes?

Look beyond the medical justifications for improving your diabetes control outlined in Chapter 1, and usually you find psychological issues that motivate your decision.

Some people strive for excellence in whatever they do and insist on the best, most exhaustive approach to any undertaking. While seeking excellence is admirable, it must be tempered by reality and not done at the expense of other aspects of your life.

To set the almost unreachable goal of totally normal glucose patterns while ignoring the rest of life seems foolish. When people try this and inevitably fail, they are often so tormented by their failure that they lose sight of the ultimate objective—good health so that they can enjoy life. Goals are admirable, but if they are not likely to be reached, be prepared to accept *and be satisfied* with something less.

Some people blame a multitude of ills—fatigue, failed interpersonal relationships, stress-induced anxiety or depression, or business difficulties—on their diabetes control. They hope intensive therapy will make things perfect again, but more often than not, their perceived shortcomings have little if anything to do with their diabetes.

Giving relentless attention to intensive therapy while ignoring the real causes for that other problem that concerns you will not make your life any better. If you undertake intensive therapy to solve a problem you think results from substandard control, be sure there really *is* a relationship between diabetes control and that issue!

Intensive diabetes therapy may also be undertaken to compensate for variations in scheduling or activity. Many people consciously or subconsciously feel that intensive therapy will allow them more latitude with their diet, timing, and activity variations.

Yes, intensive therapy provides a mechanism to adapt to life's daily variations. However, to do so takes effort, thought, and discipline. You cannot eat whenever you want and expect the intensive program to automatically fix the problem.

Intensive therapy provides people who *must* vary their meal plan, timing, or activity with the mechanism to compensate *if* they pay close attention to these variables. Otherwise, the compensatory mechanism will not work. Those who undertake intensive therapy without realizing that this effort is necessary face frustration and disappointment.

## Is intensive therapy right for you?

Intensive diabetes therapy is not for everyone. We've discussed the medical reasons for this. From the psychological standpoint, certain characteristics make for optimal intensive therapy candidates, while other characteristics foretell disaster.

As you read the discussion that follows, think about yourself honestly. Does the description sound like you? To undertake intensive diabetes therapy when you are not well suited for it is not wise. To decide against intensive therapy because you recognize some personal traits that may cause difficulty is nothing to be ashamed of. It doesn't mean you are a bad person or psychologically unbalanced; it just means that you recognize that an intensive approach to your diabetes may not have enough of a benefit to outweigh the potential problems.

## Psychological profile of an ideal intensive therapy patient

To undertake intensive diabetes therapy, you must be highly motivated and willing to perform frequent blood tests and make frequent insulin adjustments. You must be basically optimistic and able to handle adversity fairly well. You must be prepared to accept failure if it occurs, although we hope you will set realistic goals and therefore be successful!

The rigors of intensive therapy require someone just compulsive enough to perform the testing, analyze the variables, (especially eating, timing, and activity), and quantitate them and adjust them as the need arises. However, you cannot be so compulsive that your whole life becomes focused on intensive therapy, with success or failure controlling your attitudes and actions toward other goals in your life.

There will be successful days and unsuccessful days. While you need to assess why these have occurred and act to maximize the successful days, if you excessively ruminate over your failures, you will become overburdened testing and assessing to the exclusion of living and achieving other goals. Also, you must be able to accept that on occasion you will "burn out" and get sick of intensive therapy. You must be able to slack off on the rigors of intensive therapy for a period of time to give yourself a mental break.

You must be able to think independently and make decisions with confidence, yet also have enough insight into your abilities to know your limitations and to call for help when needed. You must be a strong and self-assured individual so that when testing or scheduling requirements affect your activities with others, you handle your own needs without giving in to group pressures. You must feel comfortable with, and be able to educate those around you about why you are testing so frequently. You should feel comfortable in your ability to make appropriate adaptations so you can participate in social activities you enjoy.

You need to be comfortable with the visible signs that you have diabetes—testing your blood in public, giving yourself injections, or wearing a pump. It is important that you fully integrate your diabetes into your lifestyle. *You cannot resent your diabetes.* You cannot deny it or ignore it to the point of harming yourself. You must feel committed to the importance of diabetes treatment. With the rigors of intensive therapy, if you don't believe in what you are doing, your enthusiasm will fade rapidly.

*Trust* is another important attribute of an ideal candidate for intensive diabetes therapy. You need support from those close to you—your spouse, other relatives, friends, and coworkers. Your family members may need support from your health care team as they cope with their fears of hypoglycemia or as they work through the problems they may have that result in criticizing you and how you are handling your intensive therapy. You must trust that your family's support will be there if you need it—there to support you emotionally and there to help out should you encounter treatment difficulties.

You also must trust your health care team, who work with you, advise you, and guide you. Think about what they recommend, be sure that you agree with it, feel comfortable questioning them about things you don't understand or don't agree with. But also feel comfortable that they can give you the proper advice and guide you correctly.

You should also be a person who follows through with whatever you undertake. You should not start an intensive diabetes program thinking it is something to dabble in. Certainly, intensive therapy can be abandoned if desired, but to succeed, your heart must be in it and you should not *plan* on backing out with the first frustration.

Finally, you must have good overall psychological health. People who have suffered from depressive or anxiety disorders may have these reactivated by the rigors of intensive therapy. Intensive therapy is a psychological stress, and anyone who feels he or she cannot handle such stress should consider "intensifying" their current treatment program, perhaps, but should probably not embark on a true intensive program.

## Psychological aspects of using intensive therapy

Once intensive therapy has started, there are a number of psychological pitfalls to avoid.

The biggest challenge is to recognize the program's limitations, if you fall short of your original goals. Technology has still not developed methods to completely normalize blood glucose metabolism for those with insulin dependent diabetes.

All intensive therapies attempt to mimic normal insulin action, but their success is variable, so, it may become necessary to accept something less than your initial goals. You must try to accept it without anger toward the health care team for failing you, without frustration toward medical science for being inept in its research, and, most importantly, without blaming yourself for somehow not living up to your medical needs or expectations.

Beware of the opposite situation as well: When the therapy is so good you may be driven to do better and better, to have lower and lower blood glucose levels. To struggle with high or unstable sugars when everyone sings the virtues of normal glucose levels and then to suddenly acquire the means to approach normalized patterns can be thrilling.

### Concerns around hypoglycemia

Beware! The goal may be *normal* sugars, but you must also *achieve them safely!* People have encountered serious difficulty or even death when, driven by a fear of high sugars or thrill over the ability to normalize them, they try to achieve lower and lower glucose levels. With lower glucose levels, the danger of hypoglycemia increases.

Some people using intensive diabetes therapy lose the ability to sense the early warning symptoms of an approaching reaction ("hypoglycemic unawareness"). The first sign of a reaction may be confusion or even unconsciousness, which can be dangerous, as well as frightening to both family and friends. It is important to work with the health care team to reduce both consequences and fears of hypoglycemic unawareness. Set reasonable and safe goals, and stick to them!

### You can become addicted to your success

Don't become too emotionally attached to your diabetes treatment. Yes, you are *physiologically* dependent on your insulin treatment, but don't become *psychologically* dependent. Some people become so emotionally attached to their intensive therapy that it becomes part of their identity. While this occurs more often with pump therapy, it can occur with multiple daily injections as well.

Emotional attachments may occur because this treatment is the first that you felt comfortable with, because it provides more freedom and pleasure, or because you know that your success pleases others. A pump user might become the community celebrity, speaking at diabetes group meetings and advising other patients. Their pump is their ticket to fame. Take it away, and you take away part of their identity.

With such close attachment to your treatment program, you cannot view it objectively, and may not accept suggestions from your health care team for adjustments or change. Like any other inanimate object or concept, intensive insulin treatment programs may need to be adapted or even abandoned at some time in the future. Emotion must not stand in the way of objective treatment decisions.

## Summary

If you are currently considering intensive therapy, think about how you might handle the psychological rigors of this undertaking. Would you fall into some of the psychological traps discussed above? Could you handle the frustration of failure? Could you be objective about success?

If you are already on intensive therapy, have some of the issues discussed put into words feelings you may have wrestled with already, but had not recognized as conscious issues? By identifying some of the problems, can you now gain enough insight to find appropriate solutions? You may now realize that the mental health professional who is part of your health care team can help you deal with some of these issues.

Your health care team will help you, not just with insulin doses and algorithms, but with the psychological aspects of intensive therapy as well. The goal of therapy is not just proper glycohemoglobin levels but the quality of the life you lead.

# Chapter Eleven

# When Things Go Awry

■ How can you help yourself
when things go wrong
with your intensified or intensive
diabetes management?

Life is not always smooth sailing and you may confront urgent issues in your intensive diabetes therapy. At those times, check this chapter for a helpful approach to some of the most common "emergencies." While this chapter is not a substitute for reading the whole book or seeking the advice of your health care team, in a pinch, it is a start.

But *be prepared!* Review the potential problems and solutions *before* they occur. Make advance preparations where indicated and discuss them with your health care team. Make notes in the margins, if necessary. Then, when trouble strikes, you will be prepared.

Needless to say, if in doubt about any of these problems, contact your health care team as soon as possible!

### Sick days

**Question: I'm on an MDI program and feel I'm getting "flu" symptoms and maybe the start of a fever. What should I do?**

1. Monitor your blood glucose *and* test your urine for ketones at least every 4 hours, around the clock. Set an alarm during the night. (Ketones plus a high sugar suggest a more urgent need for extra insulin.)

2. Always take your usual daily dose of insulin. *Never omit it.* You still need insulin, *even if you are unable to eat,* but in this circumstance, you may need to be in a hospital.

3. Before you get sick, discuss with your health care team what your sick-day insulin protocol should be. The protocol suggested below is a guide, but a personalized program is better.

4. When your blood glucose/urine ketone tests show a *blood glucose value of 240 to 400 mg/dl and the urine shows no ketones,*

take 10 percent of your total daily insulin dose as regular insulin. Calculate this total by adding all of your usual insulin doses together. Use the regular insulin dose on your algorithm for a blood glucose range 100 to 150 mg/dl (or the approximate equivalent) for this calculation.

5. At the time of a blood glucose/urine ketone test, if the *blood glucose value is over 400 mg/dl with or without ketones, or if it is over 240 with ketones,* take an extra, or booster, dose of 20 percent of your total daily insulin dose in the form of regular insulin.

6. If this coincides with a scheduled time to take an insulin dose, calculate your regular insulin dose based on your usual algorithm, and add the 10 percent or 20 percent booster dose to the dose of regular that you would take based on the algorithm.

7. Do not take extra insulin for blood glucose values less than 240 mg/dl even if ketones are present in the urine. Just follow your algorithm.

8. Take liquids every hour. Food suggestions for sick days are listed on page 160. If you are unable to take liquids because of nausea or vomiting, contact your health care team.

9. Rest and keep warm. Do not exercise. Have someone take care of you.

10. If you are vomiting, in pain, or cannot control your blood glucose levels, contact your physician immediately.

## Sick day food suggestions

(Each item equals 15 grams of carbohydrate)

| | |
|---|---|
| Applesauce (sweetened) | 1/2 cup |
| Apple juice | 1/2 cup |
| Baked custard | 1/2 cup |
| Coke® syrup | 1 1/2 tablespoons |
| Cooked cereal | 1/2 cup |
| Cream soups | 1 cup |
| Eggnog | 1/2 cup |
| Fruit yogurt | 1/3 cup |
| Frozen yogurt | |
|  –on a stick | 1 bar |
|  –from container | 1/3 cup |
| Grape juice | 3 ounces |
| Honey | 3 teaspoons |
| Hershey's ™ syrup | 2 tablespoons |
| LifeSavers® | 7 |
| Milk shake | 1/4 cup |
| Popsicle® (twin-pop) | 1 |
| Pudding (sweetened) | 1/4 cup |
| Regular ice cream | 1/2 cup |
| Regular JELL-O® | 1/3 cup |
| Regular soft drinks | 1/3 cup |
| Saltines® | 6 |
| Sherbert | 1/4 cup |
| Toast | 1 slice |

**Question: I use ultralente before breakfast and before supper and regular before each meal, and I need to follow sick day rules. How would I calculate the 10 percent and 20 percent booster rules for insulin with this sort of program?**

1. Follow all of the rules for *when* to take an extra dose discussed in the previous question.

2. Boosters for this type of ultralente/regular program should be given as *regular insulin* only.

3. Continue the same dose of ultralente without any change, unless your health care team has instructed you to do otherwise.

4. Calculate your total daily dose by adding the regular insulin doses for glucose ranges of 100 to 150 mg/dl (or the equivalent) *plus* the two injections of ultralente.

5. Determine whether you need 10 percent or 20 percent boosters as in the first question above.

**Question: I use a pump for my diabetes treatment and feel that I'm getting the "flu" with typical symptoms and maybe the start of a fever. What should I do?**

1. Be sure that you are testing for blood glucose levels *and* for urine ketones at least every 4 hours, around the clock, just as you would with an MDI program.

2. Always take your usual daily dose of insulin. Never omit it, even if you are unable to eat.

3. Before you ever get sick, discuss with your health care team what your catch-up insulin plan should be. The plan suggested below is a guide, but a personalized program is better.

4. While sick, increase your basal rate by 50 percent if your blood glucose level is above 240 mg/dl, whether or not you have ketones present in your urine. Thus, if your basal rate was 1.2 units per hour, it should be increased to 1.8 units per hour (1.2 + 0.6 = 1.8).

5. At the time of a blood glucose/urine ketone test, if the *blood glucose value is 240 to 400 mg/dl and the urine shows no ketones,* take 10 percent of your total daily insulin dose as a bolus of regular insulin (see item 7 below).

6. At the time of a blood glucose/urine ketone test, if the *blood glucose value is over 400 mg/dl with or without ketones, or if it is over 240 with ketones,* take 20 percent of your total daily insulin dose as a bolus of regular insulin (see item 7 below).

7. To calculate your total daily insulin dose, add the total insulin that you receive each day through the basal insulin infusion to the sum of the regular insulin boluses that you would give for blood glucose values in the 100 to 150 mg/dl range (or a close equivalent range) before each meal and each snack. (For example: your basal is 1.0 unit/hour, or 24 units per day. For glucose levels 100 to 150 mg/dl, you would take 6 units before breakfast, 4 before lunch, 5 before supper, and 1 before bedtime snack, for a total bolus quantity of 16. 24 + 16 = 40. 10 percent of this is 4 units, 20 percent is 8 units.)

8. If the high blood glucose test coincides with a scheduled time to take an insulin dose, calculate your regular insulin dose based on your usual algorithm, and add the 10 percent or 20 percent incremental dose to the dose of regular that you would take for your bolus based on the algorithm.

9. Do not take extra insulin for blood glucose values under 240 mg/dl even if ketones are present in the urine.

10. Take liquids every hour. Food suggestions for sick days are listed on page 160. If you are unable to take liquids because of nausea or vomiting, contact your health care team.

11. Rest and keep warm. Do not exercise. Have someone take care of you.

12. If in doubt about the pump's effectiveness in bringing down your blood glucose levels, or if it is actually failing to do so, use injected insulin and your off-pump insulin dose.

13. If you are vomiting, in pain, or cannot control your blood glucose levels, contact your physician immediately.

### Question: What should I do if I can't keep food down?

The inability to hold down food, and especially solids *and* liquids, is a true emergency for someone with insulin dependent diabetes. You may need to be given intravenous fluid and glucose.

Call your health care team immediately. If they are unavailable, or you are away from home, go to a hospital emergency room.

Do not be alarmed if the doctors in the emergency room are not familiar with your insulin treatment program. What you need is the intravenous treatment and enough insulin at that moment to manage your diabetes. The MDI or pump program can be put on hold temporarily.

### Question: Are there other situations when I should think of following my sick day protocol?

Blood glucose levels can be high because of any stress to the body. Think of sick day rules with any infection (skin, vaginal, bladder, etc.), injury or trauma, or serious medical condition such as a heart attack or stroke.

Of course, for some of these, you would be in a hospital setting fairly quickly, and the doctors should be watching over your diabetes. However, they may be concentrating on your other problems, particularly if they are not trained in internal medicine and are, perhaps, treating your broken bones or acute appendicitis. Keep informed about your blood sugars, and, if they are very high, ask your doctors to consult a specialist in diabetes management (a diabetologist, endocrinologist, or internist).

**Question: I'm using the pump. I'm not sick, but my blood glucose tests are suddenly high. What should I do?**

If a pump malfunctions, very high blood sugar levels can result rapidly, leading to diabetic ketoacidosis. Therefore, any unexplained high blood glucose test is a potential danger, and two in a row warrant thought and attention.

Use the following checklist as a guide to various possible explanations for elevated sugars. (It is always a good idea to review this list in advance with your health care team; they may want to add or delete certain items.) Many of the suggestions and questions outlined below may require discussions with your health care team anyway.

A. *Have you been eating more food?*
   If so, do you need a further adjustment in your program to compensate for increased eating, or do you need a diet review to get back in the proper eating plan?

B. *Have you been getting less exercise?*
   If this is permanent or semipermanent, should you adjust your algorithm?

C. *Are you coming down with a cold or flu?*
   If so, time will tell. Rule out other possible explanations, and then, if your algorithm is not bringing you back into line,

take about 10 percent more insulin in your boluses for a day or so. If no cold or flu appears or if you are spilling ketones, call your health care team.

D. *If you are a woman, are you about to have your period?*
You may want to talk to your health care team about future compensatory adjustments in your basal rates or bolus doses before your periods.

E. *Have you forgotten to take your boluses?*
Why are you forgetting?

F. *Is your syringe empty?*
Check and refill if necessary. Why did it get empty? Think about your refilling routine and check it more often if necessary.

G. *Is the pump programmed correctly?*
Check programming against what you are supposed to be getting and be sure it's correct. Is the pump in "suspend" mode?

H. *Is there a leak or a blockage in the infusion set?* ★
Check syringe and infusion set carefully. Was the tubing kinked or twisted? Is there blood in the tubing? Is the stress loop adequate?

I. *Is there air in the infusion set?* ★
Check syringe and infusion set.

J. *Is the insulin potent?*
Has the insulin passed its expiration date? Has the insulin been exposed to extremes of temperature (over 90 degrees at all,

★*As a general rule, it is a good idea to change your infusion set, syringe, and insertion site even if a leak or blockage is not clearly noticed. Blockages may be more common if you have been in a warm environment.*

over 75 degrees for extended periods, or freezing)? Has the loaded pump been exposed to freezing or excessively warm temperatures? Have you been using insulin that is proper for pumps?

*K. Is the problem at the infusion site?*＊
Examine your infusion site carefully for inflammation or infection. Check for hypertrophy (bulging) or atrophy (wasting) of the insertion area; either can affect insulin absorption. Was the needle inserted properly?

*L. Are the batteries dead?*
Check them! Are you changing batteries often enough or is there a problem with the recharging?

*M. Is the pump mechanism working properly?*
Remove the needle and shoot a bolus into the air with the pump. If no insulin comes out, try a new infusion set. If insulin still doesn't come out and all of the other above issues have been ruled out, assume the pump is malfunctioning and use an off-pump insulin dose until you can contact your health care team or the pump manufacturer service representative.

Once the pump appears to be working properly again, continue to wear it and receive your *sick day basal rate* through the pump. However, give the bolus insulin doses subcutaneously *by syringe* until blood glucose levels come to below 240 mg/dl. Only then should you return to your usual basal and take the bolus doses using the pump.

---

＊ *As a general rule, it is a good idea to change your infusion set, syringe, and insertion site even if a problem at the infusion site is not clearly noticeable.*

*If in doubt, use the off-pump insulin dose and inject all insulin by syringe until you can contact your health care team and determine what the problem is. If you cannot bring your blood glucose levels down under 400 mg/dl after 24 hours, or if they are persistently over 240 with ketones, contact your health care team.*

### Question: I use a pump. How do I know what my off-pump insulin dose should be in case I need to go back to injected insulin?

As a general rule, always determine your off-pump dose before actually needing it. This dose should be reviewed with your health care team. However, if you have not done this, and you need such a dose immediately, the following guidelines give two ways such a dose can be calculated. Review the dose at the earliest possible time with your health care team.

A. Add up the total number of basal units of insulin delivered in 24 hours. This is the total basal dose.

  1. Take 60 percent of the total basal dose as NPH or lente before breakfast.

  2. Take 40 percent of the total basal dose as NPH or lente at bedtime.

B. Follow the pump algorithms for regular insulin doses before breakfast, lunch, and supper.

C. Alternatively, calculate your total daily dose of basal plus regular doses for glucose ranges in the 100 to 150 range. Take two-thirds of this as NPH or lente, 60 percent of this total before breakfast, and 40 percent at bedtime. Take the remaining one-third as regular, 60 percent before breakfast and 40 percent before supper.

**Question: I have developed a red, sore area at the insertion site for my pump infusion set or at the site of an insulin injection. What should I do?**

While such occurrences are relatively rare, they do happen and may represent a skin infection at that location. The most common cause of this is having left the needle in too long. These sites may require treatment with antibiotics and might even need to be drained surgically. Infections often cause elevated blood glucose levels as well. Contact your health care team. Until treatment can be started, watch your glucose levels carefully, and do not hesitate to use sick day rules if needed.

**Question: I use a pump and have had a severe hypoglycemic reaction. I'm now better, but how should I determine what caused this reaction and how to help prevent future ones?**

Ask yourself the following questions:

A. *Did you eat less food than usual?*
   Do you need to review your meal plan with a dietitian?

B. *Were you more active than usual?*
   At the time of the reaction? During a period of up to 12 or more hours before the reaction (remember the lag effect)? Review adjustments in food and insulin for exercise with your health care team.

C. *Did you take a larger bolus of insulin because of anticipated increased food intake that either did not actually occur or did occur but at a lesser quantity or later time than expected?*

D. *Did you program the pump properly?*
   Check pump programming

E. *Have you consumed any alcoholic beverages in the last 12 hours?*
   If so, avoid any alcoholic beverages until you have a chance to
   review with your health care team the effects of alcohol on
   diabetes control.

F. *Had you disconnected the infusion set from the syringe just before the*
   *reaction?*
   Gravity can pull insulin in the infusion set into your body if
   you are not careful. Review disconnection technique with
   your health care team.

*If you have no obvious answer, consider removing your pump and using your*
*off-pump insulin dose until you can contact your health care team.*

**Question: I had been doing well with my intensive diabetes**
**program, and then all of a sudden, things fell apart! I'm now**
**having reactions and lots of high sugar readings. What do I**
**do?**

Intensive diabetes therapy requires a very precise balance of the
many factors that affect blood glucose levels. Although the major
categories of eating, insulin, activity, timing, and physical stresses
usually cover most of the issues, it is sometimes difficult to recognize
the precise role each may be playing, and other, less obvious factors
may be difficult to identify. In addition, insulin requirements may
simply change over time as you age.

Anyone who has read this book and undertakes intensive therapy
should, by now, know what to think about when sugars go awry:

• Check food quantity and timing.

• Check activity amount and timing.

• Look at reactions and rebounds that may not have produced
  obvious symptoms.

- Make sure the insulin is potent and is getting into you the way that it is supposed to.

- Make sure there is no physical stress, such as illness, infection, or injury.

However, exploring these issues may not yield an obvious explanation. Frequently, you need to review things in detail with your health care team to either discover what the problem is, or figure out how to uncover it. Before calling the team (assuming the reactions or highs are not acutely dangerous), consider a few things:

- Review the issues raised by the other questions in this chapter.

- Has your routine been interrupted or altered? It is not uncommon for a change to affect any of the diabetes control factors. This may occur during or after a vacation, with the change of seasons, or with a new job.

- Try reducing the insulin doses (unless your sugars are all high). You still may be having unrecognized reactions and rebounds. Patterns can be clearer with slightly high sugar levels.

- Are you really following your routine as carefully as you should? Be honest with yourself!

- Has this happened before? It is not uncommon for people on intensive therapy who are watching glucose levels quite closely to have good periods and bad periods for reasons that may not be entirely clear. You may just need to wait out the bad period.

Once you have thought about these issues, and perhaps tried a few maneuvers, call your health care team for help. Doing this homework beforehand can help them help you!

**Question: I've had it! Intensive therapy is too intense and I cannot deal with it any more. Help! What can I do?**

Clearly, these emotions are not uncommon when you use intensive diabetes therapy. If you didn't feel this way on occasion, you wouldn't be normal! So you know you are normal. That doesn't make the frustration go away! Well, there are things you can do that will help.

Start by talking with your diabetes health care team. Depending on the reason for starting intensive diabetes therapy, you might be able to slack off a little or even stop intensive therapy for a while. Of course, if you are using intensive therapy because conventional therapy was unsafe or ineffective, the ability to lessen your grip on intensity may be limited.

You may want to discuss your frustrations with the health care team, and perhaps a mental health professional. Targeting aspects of intensive therapy that are particularly upsetting or frustrating may help your team make treatment adjustments that are easier for you to live with. Don't just wallow in your misery! Talk things over.

For some, it may be possible to take a vacation from intensive therapy. Discuss this with your health care team to determine alternative insulin doses and testing programs, and determine when you may resume intensive therapy.

## Summary

In general, when problems arise, good common sense and a solid understanding of diabetes self-treatment are often your best guides. When in doubt call for help. Frequently, your telephone can get you the information you need. If all else fails, seek care, nearby if the problem is urgent or serious. Knowing the limitations of what you can handle and what requires help from others may be the difference between serious consequences and a rapid return to good health.

# INTENSIFIED CONVENTIONAL TREATMENT PROGRAMS

Guidelines for establishing an intensified conventional treatment program using a morning mixed dose of regular and intermediate (NPH or lente), presupper regular, and bedtime intermediate (NPH or lente) insulin.

**Note:** These guidelines are general and are included to give an example of how an intensified conventional program could be set up. They are not the only way to set up such a program. Your health care team may approach the establishment of this program in another way.

**Under no circumstances should anyone use these guidelines to switch treatment programs without the guidance of a physician who is trained in diabetes treatment and/or a diabetes health care team.**

- Establish your total daily insulin dose. This can be determined either by totalling the present insulin doses or calculating the total dose based on body weight. (Approximately 0.5 unit per kilogram of body weight is often used.)

- The intermediate insulin doses are about two-thirds of this total daily dose.

- Regular insulin makes up the other one-third. This amount of regular insulin is often divided so two-thirds of the total regular is given before breakfast and one-third before supper.

Since this is an estimate, round up or down when fractions occur. Then adjust the insulin based on blood glucose monitoring.

```
                    E X A M P L E
```

**Calculating a dose for a three-injection split-mix program**
Your calculated total daily dose is 36 units.
         —Your three-injection, split-mix insulin doses would be:

| Insulin | Given as: | Represents about: |
|---|---|---|
| 24 units | Total daily NPH or lente | 67% of daily total insulin |
| 12 units | Total daily regular | 33% of daily total insulin |
| | **Dosage breakdown** | |
| 16 units | Prebreakfast NPH or lente insulin | 67% of daily total of NPH or lente |
| 8 units | Prebreakfast regular insulin for glucose values of 100-150 mg/dl | 67% of daily total of regular |
| 4 units | Presupper regular insulin for glucose values of 100-150 mg/dl | 33% of daily total of regular |
| 8 units | Bedtime NPH or lente insulin | 33% of daily total of NPH or lente |

An algorithm is then designed by increasing the dose (usually by 1 unit) for every 50 points above 150 mg/dl and decreasing the dose for every 50 points below 100 mg/dl.

## Well day insulin adjustments for a premeal regular and bedtime intermediate insulin program

Before adjusting insulin, you must be:
    —Following your meal plan
    —Using your testing equipment correctly
    —Not sick
    —Sure you are not having hypoglycemic reactions and rebounding.

Be sure you have discussed your initial blood glucose goals with your health care team and that they are safe and realistic. For people seeking DCCT level control, your goal inevitably will become lower (eventually) than what is listed here.Generally, initial goals established to help you get underway will be:    Fasting          100 to 150 mg/dl

                                      Premeals and bedtime   100 to 150 mg/dl

However, your goals may be different. Also, the frequency of blood glucose test results outside these limits or the duration of time with tests out of these limits may vary from person to person. Be sure you have discussed when to begin "well day adjustments" with your health care team.

## For high blood glucose levels

• *High fasting values*

After four days in a row of high fasting blood glucose test results (whatever your health care team defines as high for you), check your blood glucose level at 2 A.M. to help determine the cause:

—If the 2 A.M. test is low (suggested by a value less than 100 mg/dl) the high fasting test results may be due to rebound. Decrease the bedtime intermediate insulin dose by one unit.

—If the 2 A.M. test is high (100 mg/dl or more) the high fasting test result may be due to insufficient insulin action overnight. Increase the bedtime intermediate insulin dose by 1 unit.

Wait at least *four days* between each change in the bedtime intermediate insulin dose.

• *For high premeal test results,* adjust the regular insulin sliding scale or the morning intermediate insulin doses as follows:

—For prelunch high blood sugars (whatever your health care team has determined for you) increase the morning scale by 1 unit.

—For presupper high blood sugars (whatever your team has defined as high for you), increase the morning intermediate insulin by 1 to 2 units (as instructed by your team). Beware of early onset of intermediate insulin causing hypoglycemia before lunch. The prebreakfast regular scale may need to be adjusted or a larger morning snack may be needed.

• *For high blood sugars at bedtime* (as determined by your health care team), increase the suppertime scale by 1 unit.

Alternatively, if the interval between supper and bedtime is long (4 to 5 hours or more) a small (2 to 3 unit) dose of intermediate insulin could be added to the suppertime dose of regular.

Wait two days minimum between each adjustment in the sliding scale algorithm.

## For low blood sugars

If your blood sugar is low (below whatever threshold your team has set for you) for *three days in a row*, at the same time of the day and without symptoms of an insulin reaction, increases in activity, or decreases in food, you should **decrease** the appropriate insulin as noted above under the high blood sugar section.

Wait *two days* between each adjustment in your sliding scales and four days between each adjustment in the bedtime intermediate insulin dose.

If you have an unexplained hypoglycemic insulin reaction (with blood glucose under 60 mg/dl that you can't explain by a decrease in the food you've eaten, an increase in activity, or an error in your dose) *decrease* the appropriate insulin the *very next day,* as noted above.

## Sick day guidelines

- Booster injections of extra regular insulin are usually needed in addition to your usual insulin doses during the day. *(Blood glucose values should be at or higher than 240 mg/dl when using booster rules.)*

- Booster injections are given every 3 to 4 hours based on blood glucose testing and urine ketones. They are given as regular insulin only.

- Continue the same doses of intermediate insulin without any change.

- If you need to use the sick day booster more than twice, you should contact your health care team.

- Stop using the sick day booster when your blood sugar comes down below 240 mg/dl.

- Ketones take longer to leave the body, so you may see ketones in the urine the next day. Drink extra fluids to help flush out the ketones.

- If you CAN eat, drink plenty of water or sugar-free beverages, about one cup each hour, and follow your usual meal plan.

- If you CAN'T eat, every other hour while you're awake drink one cup of fluid with sugar, such as regular soda, popsicles, ice cream, or lemonade.

- If you have nausea or are vomiting and are unable to hold down either food or drink, call your physician immediately.

- Rest

- Treat the illness appropriately. If unsure, contact your physician for advice.

**Determining your sick day booster dose of regular insulin based on your blood glucose and urine ketone testing every 3 to 4 hours**

—Total up the daily dose of insulin, both intermediate and regular insulin, needed for a blood glucose level of 100 to 150 mg/dl.

— If you are sick with a blood glucose over 240 mg/dl but with no urine ketones, take 10% of this quantity as your booster dose of regular insulin.

— If you are sick with a blood glucose over 240 mg/dl and do have ketones in your urine or if the glucose is over 400 mg/dl regardless of whether ketones are present, take 20% of this quantity as your booster dose of regular insulin.

## E X A M P L E

**Calculating sick day insulin booster
for a three-injection split-mix program**

—**Your usual three-injection, split-mix insulin doses are:**

| Insulin | Given as: |
|---|---|
| 20 units | Prebreakfast NPH or lente insulin |
| 6 units | Prebreakfast regular insulin for glucose values of 100–150 mg/dl |
| 6 units | Presupper regular insulin for glucose values of 100–150 mg/dl |
| 8 units | Bedtime NPH or lente insulin |
| **40 units** | **Total daily insulin dose** |

**Your sick day booster doses would be:**

| | |
|---|---|
| 4 units | Regular insulin for a catch-up dose of 10% of daily total |
| 8 units | Regular insulin for a catch-up dose of 20% of daily total |

If this dose comes due at the time a routine premeal regular insulin dose is due, add the booster quantity of regular insulin to the insulin dictated by your algorithm.

For example, using the above insulin doses, if the blood glucose level is 365 mg/dl before breakfast, with positive ketones, and the algorithm shows that 10 units of regular insulin should be given, the sick day doses would be 10 + 8 (20% booster) for a total of 18 units of regular insulin.

**Other important information about intensified conventional insulin therapy**

- Never adjust more than one insulin at a time.

- Don't make more than two adjustments without checking with your health care team, unless otherwise instructed.

- Check your weight. It is very easy to gain weight using this or any form of intensified diabetes therapy. If you do gain weight, review your meal plan with your dietitian.

- Snacking may be necessary with this type of insulin treatment program. Snacks should be eaten at the time of the daytime insulin peaks, especially if you have been active. This would include late morning, late afternoon, and bedtime.

- Your insulin can become weak if left out of the refrigerator for too long. Do not leave insulin out of the refrigerator for more than 30 days. (Nonrefrigeration for travel should not be a problem.)

# ULTRALENTE

### Guidelines for establishing an ultralente/regular program

**NOTE:** These guidelines are general and are included as an example of how an ultralente program could be set up. They are not the only way to determine an ultralente/regular program. Your health care team may approach this program in another way.

**Under no circumstances should anyone use these guidelines to switch to an ultralente program without the guidance of a physician who is trained in diabetes treatment and/or a diabetes health care team.**

- Establish the total daily insulin dose, either by totalling the present insulin doses or calculating it based on the body weight (approximately 0.5 unit per kilogram of body weight is often used).

- Ultralente is about 50% of this total daily dose. For a two injection program, half of this (25% of the *total* daily dose) is given before breakfast, and half before supper.

- Regular insulin makes up the other 50% of the total daily dose of insulin. It is often divided among the premeal doses so that, for a blood glucose value of 100 to 150 mg/dl, the dose makes up the following percents:

| Percent of total daily dose of REGULAR INSULIN | | Percent of total daily dose of ALL INSULINS (R+U) |
|---|---|---|
| Prebreakfast: | 40% | 20% |
| Prelunch: | 30% | 15% |
| Presupper: | 30% | 15% |

Since this is an estimated dose, round up or down when fractions occur and then adjust based on actual test result.

---

**E X A M P L E**

**Calculating a dose for an ultralente/regular program**
Your calculated total daily dose is 40 units.

**—Your ultralente/regular insulin doses would be:**

| Insulin | Given as: | Represents about: |
|---------|-----------|-------------------|
| 20 units | Total daily ultralente | 50% of daily total insulin |
| 20 units | Total daily regular | 50% of daily total insulin |

**Dosage breakdown**

| | | |
|---------|-----------|-------------------|
| 10 units | Prebreakfast ultralente | 50% of daily total of ultralente |
| 10 units | Presupper ultralente insulin | 50% of daily total of ultralente |
| 8 units | Prebreakfast regular insulin for glucose values of 100–150 mg/dl | 40% of daily total of regular |
| 6 units | Prelunch regular insulin for glucose values of 100–150 mg/dl | 30% of daily total of regular |
| 6 units | Presupper regular insulin for glucose values of 100–150 mg/dl | 30% of daily total of regular |

An algorithm is then designed by increasing the dose (usually by one unit) for every 50 points above 150 mg/dl, and decreasing by every 50 points below 100 mg/dl.

There is no need to change the previous insulin dose ahead of time. Ultralente can be started the day the decision is made to use this insulin.

## Well day insulin adjustments of an ultralente program (ultralente before breakfast and supper, regular before meals)

Before adjusting insulin, you must be:
—Following your meal plan
—Using your testing equipment correctly
—Not sick
—Sure you're not having hypoglycemic reactions and rebounding.

Be sure you have discussed your blood glucose goals with your health care team and that they are safe and realistic. For people seeking DCCT level control, your goal inevitably will, over time and through experience, become lower than what is listed here. Generally, initial goals established to help you get underway will be:

> Fasting:                100-150 mg/dl
> Premeals and bedtime:   100-150 mg/dl

However, your goals may be different. The frequency of blood glucose test results outside these limits, or the duration of time with tests out of these limits, may vary from individual to individual. Be sure you have discussed with your health care team when you should begin "well day adjustments."

### For high blood glucose levels

- *High fasting values.*—After *4 days* in a row of high fasting blood glucose test results (whatever your health care team defines as high), verify by checking a blood glucose level at 2 A.M..

  —If the 2 A.M. test result is low (suggested by a value of 100 mg/dl or less), the high fasting test result may be caused by rebound. *Decrease* the ultralente doses by 1 unit each.

  —If the 2 A.M. test result is high (at or above 100 mg/dl), the high fasting test result may be due to insufficient insulin action overnight. *Increase* the ultralente doses by 1 unit each.

NOTE: The dose changes should be for each dose of ultralente. If you take one injection of ultralente, then the change is 1 unit for that one dose. If you take two daily ultralente injections, you change each dose by 1 unit, for a total of 2 units per day, and so on.

**183**

Wait *at least 4 days* between each change in the ultralente dose.

- *For high premeal test results,* adjust the regular insulin algorithm:

    —*For prelunch high blood sugars* (whatever parameters your health care team has determined for you), increase the morning scale by 1 unit.

    —*For presupper high blood sugars* (whatever parameters your health care team has determined for you), increase the lunchtime scale by 1 unit.

    —*For bedtime high blood sugars* (whatever parameters your health care team has determined for you), increase the suppertime scale by 1 unit.

Wait *two* days minimum between each adjustment in the sliding scale algorithm. You may be instructed to wait longer.

### For low blood glucose levels

*If your blood sugar is low* (below whatever level your health care team has set as your lower goal) for *three days in a row,* at the same time of day, without symptoms of an insulin reaction or explanations related to a temporary decrease in your eating or increase in your activity, *decrease* the appropriate insulin as noted under the "high blood sugar" section above.

Wait *two days* between each adjustment in your algorithm and *four days* between each adjustment in the ultralente dose.

If you have an unexplained hypoglycemic insulin reaction (a blood glucose level under 60 mg/dl that is not due to a decrease in food or an increase in activity, or an error in your insulin dose), *decrease* the appropriate insulin the *very next day,* as noted above.

Once your ultralente program is working well, you and your health care team may wish to adjust your targeted blood sugar goals.

## Ultralente sick day guidelines

- Booster injections of extra regular insulin are usually needed in addition to your usual insulin doses during the day.
- Blood glucose values should be at or above 240 mg/dl when using booster rules.
- Booster injections are given every *3 to 4 hours*. They are given as *regular* insulin only.
- Continue the same dose of ultralente without any change.
- If you need to use the sick day booster more than twice, you should contact your health care team.
- Stop using the sick day booster when your blood sugar comes down below 240 mg/dl.
- Ketones take longer to leave the body, so you may see ketones in the urine the next day. Drink extra fluids to help flush out the ketones.
- If you *CAN* eat, drink plenty of water or sugar-free beverages, about one cup each hour, and follow your usual meal plan.
- If you *CAN'T* eat, every *other* hour while you are awake drink one cup of fluid with sugar, such as regular soda, popsicles, ice cream, or lemonade.
- If you have nausea or are vomiting, and are unable to hold down either food or drink, call your physician immediately.
- Rest
- Treat the illness appropriately. If unsure, contact your physician.

### Determining your sick day booster dose of regular insulin

- Total up your daily dose of insulin, both ultralente and the dose of regular for a blood glucose level of 100 to 150 mg/dl.
- If you are sick with a blood glucose over 240 mg/dl but with no urine ketones, take 10% of your total daily dose as your booster dose of regular insulin.
- If you are sick with a blood glucose over 240 mg/dl and do have ketones in your urine, or if the glucose is over 400 mg/dl regardless of whether ketones are present in the urine, take 20% of your total daily dose as your booster dose of regular insulin.

---

### E X A M P L E

Calculating sick day insulin booster
for an ultralente/regular insulin program
— Your usual ultralente/regular insulin doses are:

| Insulin | Given as: |
|---|---|
| 12 units | Prebreakfast ultralente |
| 12 units | Presupper ultralente |
| 7 units | Prebreakfast regular insulin for glucose values of 100–150 mg/dl |
| 4 units | Prelunch regular insulin for glucose values of 100–150 mg/dl |
| 5 units | Presupper regular insulin for glucose values of 100–150 mg/dl |
| **40 units** | **Total daily insulin dose** |

Your sick day booster doses would be:

| | |
|---|---|
| 4 units | Regular insulin for a catch-up dose of 10% of daily total |
| 8 units | Regular insulin for a catch-up dose of 20% of daily total |

---

## Switching from an ultralente/regular program to a program using regular and NPH or lente

### Switching to NPH or lente but retaining the regular insulin algorithm

Calculate the total daily dose of ultralente insulin (the basal insulin dose) and give this total as NPH or lente, divided as follows:

Morning dose: 60% of the total ultralente dose

Evening dose: 40% of the total ultralente dose (before supper)

### Switching to NPH or lente using a split mix instead of the algorithm

— Calculate the total daily dose of insulin by adding up the doses of ultralente and regular insulin as determined by the adjustment algorithm for a blood glucose value of 100 to 150 mg/dl.

— Two-thirds of this total will be given as NPH or lente.

—One-third of this total will be given as regular.

—Divide the total number of units to be given as NPH or lente so two-thirds are given before breakfast, and one-third is given at suppertime or bedtime.

— Divide the total number of units to be given as regular insulin so that two-thirds are given before breakfast, and one-third is given at suppertime.

—Test the blood carefully and adjust the doses as needed.

## E X A M P L E

**Ultralente/regular program conversion to split-mix program**

—**Your usual ultralente/regular insulin doses are:**

| Insulin | Given as: |
|---|---|
| 10 units | Prebreakfast ultralente |
| 10 units | Presupper ultralente |
| 7 units | Regular insulin for fasting blood glucose of 100–150 mg/dl |
| 4 units | Regular insulin for prelunch blood glucose of 100–150 mg/dl |
| 5 units | Regular insulin for presupper blood glucose of 100–150 mg/dl |
| **36 units** | **Total daily insulin dose** |

**Split-Mix Program:**

| Insulin | Given as: | Represents about: |
|---|---|---|
| 24 units | Total daily NPH or lente | 67% of daily total insulin |
| 12 units | Total daily regular | 33% of daily total insulin |

### Dosage breakdown

| Insulin | Given as: | Represents about: |
|---|---|---|
| 16 units | Morning NPH or lente | 67% of daily NPH or lente |
| 8 units | Suppertime or bedtime NPH or lente | 33% of daily NPH or lente |
| 8 units | Morning regular | 67% of total daily regular |
| 4 units | Suppertime regular insulin | 33% of total daily regular |

Algorithmic adjustments of the prebreakfast and presupper regular insulin doses can be used, as determined by your health care team.

## Other facts about ultralente programs

- Never adjust more than one insulin at a time.

- Don't make more than two adjustments without checking with your health care team unless otherwise instructed.

- To improve the absorption of ultralente, use different injection sites for morning and evening injections.

- Check your weight. It is very easy to gain weight using this or any form of intensive diabetes therapy. If you do gain weight, review your meal plan with your dietitian.

- Snacking is not routinely necessary with ultralente programs. However, snacks may be needed before or after exercise, or if your bedtime blood glucose levels is less than 200 mg/dl (or whatever value you determine should be the threshold for you).

- Your insulin can lose its stability (weaken) if left out of the refrigerator for too long a period. Do not leave the insulin out of the refrigerator for more than 30 days. It is advisable to refrigerate ultralente whenever possible. (Nonrefrigeration for travel periods should not be a problem, however.)

# TREATMENT PROGRAMS USING PREMEAL REGULAR PLUS BEDTIME INTERMEDIATE INSULIN

**NOTE:** These guidelines are general and are included as an example of how a premeal regular and bedtime intermediate program could be set up. They are not the only way to determine a premeal regular and bedtime intermediate program. Your health care team may approach the establishment of this program in another way.

**Under no circumstances should anyone use these guidelines to switch himself or herself to this intensive diabetes therapy program without the guidance of a physician who is trained in diabetes treatment and/or a diabetes health care team.**

- Establish the total daily insulin dose, either by totalling present insulin doses or calculating it based on the body weight (approximately 0.5 unit per kilogram of body weight is often used).
- Bedtime intermediate is about one-fourth to one-third of the total daily dose.
- Regular insulin makes up the other two-thirds to three-fourths of the total daily dose of insulin. It is often divided among premeal doses so that, for a blood glucose value of 100 to150 mg/dl, the dose makes up the following percents:

| Percent of total daily dose of REGULAR INSULIN | | Percent of total daily dose of ALL INSULINS (R+I) |
|---|---|---|
| Prebreakfast: | 40% | 27% |
| Prelunch: | 30% | 20% |
| Presupper: | 30% | 20% |

Since this is an estimated dose, round up or down when fractions occur and then adjust based on actual test results.

---

## E X A M P L E

**Calculating a dose for a premeal
regular/bedtime intermediate program**
  Your calculated total daily insulin dose is 36 units.

**—Your premeal regular/bedtime intermediate doses would be:**

| Insulin | Given as: | Represents about: |
|---------|-----------|-------------------|
| 12 units | Total daily NPH/lente | 33% of daily total insulin |
| 24 units | Total daily regular | 67% of daily total insulin |

### Dosage breakdown

| | | |
|---------|-----------|-------------------|
| 24 units | Bedtime intermediate insulin | 100% of daily total of intermediate |
| 10 units | Prebreakfast regular insulin for glucose values of 100-150 mg/dl | 40% of daily total of ultralente |
| 7 units | Prelunch regular insulin for glucose values of 100-150 mg/dl | 30% of daily total of regular |
| 7 units | Presupper regular insulin for glucose values of 100-150 mg/dl | 30% of daily total of regular |

An algorithm is then designed by increasing the dose (usually by 1 unit) for every 50 points above 150 mg/dl and decreasing for every 50 points below 100 mg/dl. There is no need to change the previous insulin dose ahead of time, but this program should be started in the morning rather than later in the day.

### Well day insulin adjustments of a premeal regular and bedtime intermediate insulin program

Before adjusting insulin, you must be:
  —Following your meal plan
  —Using your testing equipment correctly
  —Not sick
  —Sure you are not having hypoglycemic reactions and rebounding

Be sure you have discussed your blood glucose level goals with your health care team and that they are safe and realistic. For people seeking DCCT level control, your goal inevitably, over time and through experience, will become lower than what is listed here. Generally, initial goals established to help you get underway will be:

> Fasting: 100 to 150 mg/dl
>
> Premeals and bedtime: 100 to 150 mg/dl

However, your goals may be different. The frequency of blood glucose test results outside these limits, or the duration of time with tests out of these limits, may vary from person to person. Be sure you've discussed when you should begin "well day adjustments" with your diabetes team.

## For high blood glucose levels:

*High fasting values*—After 4 days in a row of high fasting blood glucose test results (whatever your health care team defines as high for you), verify by checking a blood glucose level at 2 A.M.

—If the 2 A.M. test result is low (100 mg/dl or less), the high fasting test result may be due to rebound. Decrease the bedtime intermediate insulin dose by 1 unit.

—If the 2 A.M. test result is high (at or above 100 mg/dl), the high fasting test result may be due to insufficient insulin action overnight. Increase the bedtime intermediate insulin dose by 1 unit.

Wait at least *4 days* between each change in the bedtime intermediate insulin dose.

• For *high premeal test results,* adjust the regular insulin sliding scale:

—*For prelunch high blood sugars* (whatever parameters your health care team has determined for you), increase the morning scale by 1 unit.

—*For presupper high blood sugars* (whatever parameters your health care team has determined for you), increase the lunchtime scale by 1 unit.

—*For bedtime high blood sugars* (whatever parameters your health care team has determined for you), increase the suppertime scale by 1 unit.

Wait *two days* minimum between each adjustment in the sliding scale algorithm.

### For low blood sugars

*If your blood sugar is low* (below whatever level your health care team has set as your lower goal) for *three days in a row,* at the same time of day, without symptoms of an insulin reaction or explanations due to a temporary decrease in your eating or increase in your activity, *decrease* the appropriate insulin as noted above under the "high blood sugar" section.

Wait *two days* between each adjustment in your sliding scales and four days between each adjustment in the bedtime intermediate insulin.

If you have an unexplained hypoglycemic insulin reaction (a blood glucose level under 60 mg/dl that you cannot explain by a decrease in food or an increase in activity, or an error in your insulin dose), *decrease* the appropriate insulin a the *very next day,* as noted above.

### Sick day guidelines for premeal regular and bedtime intermediate insulin treatment programs

- Booster injections of extra regular insulin are usually needed in addition to your usual insulin doses during the day.

- Blood glucose values should be at or above 240 mg/dl when using booster rules.

- Booster injections are given every 3 to 4 hours based on the results of blood glucose testing and urine ketone testing. They are given as regular insulin only.

- Continue the same dose of bedtime intermediate insulin without any change.

- If you need to use the sick day booster more than twice, you should contact your health care team.

- Stop using the sick day booster when your blood sugar comes down below 240 mg/dl.

- Ketones take longer to leave the body, so you may see ketones in the urine the next day. Drink extra fluids to help flush out the ketones.

- If you CAN eat, drink plenty of water or sugar-free beverages, about one cup each hour, and follow your usual meal plan.

- If you CAN'T eat, every other hour while you are awake drink one cup of fluids with sugar, such as regular soda, popsicles, ice cream, or lemonade.

- If you have nausea or are vomiting and are unable to hold down either food or drink, call your physician immediately.

- Rest

- Treat the illness appropriately. If unsure, contact your physician for advice.

### Determining your sick day booster dose of regular insulin based on your blood glucose and urine ketone testing every 3 to 4 hours

—Total up your daily dose of insulin, both bedtime intermediate and premeal regular for a blood glucose level of 100 to 150 mg/dl.

—If you are sick with a blood glucose over 240 mg/dl but with no urine ketones, take 10% of this quantity as your booster dose of regular insulin.

—If you are sick with a blood glucose over 240 mg/dl and do have ketones in your urine, take 20% of this quantity as your booster dose of regular insulin.

---

### E X A M P L E

**Calculating sick day insulin booster
for a premeal regular/bedtime intermediate insulin program**

—Your usual premeal regular and bedtime
intermediate insulin doses are:

| Insulin | Given as: |
|---|---|
| 14 units | NPH or lente at bedtime |
| 11 units | Prebreakfast regular insulin for glucose values of 100-150 mg/dl |
| 7 units | Prelunch regular insulin for glucose values of 100-150 mg/dl |
| 8 units | Presupper regular insulin for glucose values of 100-150 mg/dl |
| **40 units** | **Total daily insulin dose** |

**Your sick day booster doses would be:**

| | |
|---|---|
| 4 units | Regular insulin for a catch-up dose of 10% of daily total |
| 8 units | Regular insulin for a catch-up dose of 20% of daily total |

If this dose comes due at the time that a routine premeal regular insulin dose is due, add the booster quantity of regular insulin to the quantity of insulin dictated by the algorithm for the blood glucose level.

For example, using the above insulin doses, if the blood glucose level was 365 mg/dl with positive urine ketones before supper and the algorithm indicated that, for a 365 mg/dl glucose level, 12 units of regular insulin should be given, the sick day dose would be 12+8 (20% booster), which would equal 20 units of regular insulin.

### Switching from a premeal regular and bedtime intermediate program to a standard split-mix using regular and NPH or lente

Calculate the total daily dose of insulin by adding up the doses of bedtime intermediate and premeal regular insulin as determined by the adjustment algorithm for a blood glucose value of 100 to 150 mg/dl.

# E X A M P L E

**Premeal regular/bedtime intermediate
program conversion to split-mix program**

—Your usual premeal regular and bedtime
intermediate insulin doses are:

| Insulin | Given as: |
|---|---|
| 12 units | NPH or lente at bedtime |
| 10 units | Regular insulin for a fasting blood glucose level of 100-150 mg/dl |
| 7 units | Regular insulin for a prelunch blood glucose level of 100-150 mg/dl |
| 7 units | Regular insulin for a presupper blood glucose level of 100-150 mg/dl |
| **36 units** | **Total daily insulin dose** |

**Split-mix program**

| Insulin | Given as: | Represents about: |
|---|---|---|
| 24 units | Total daily NPH/lente | 67% of daily total insulin |
| 12 units | Total daily regular | 33% of daily total insulin |

### Dosage breakdown

| | | |
|---|---|---|
| 16 units | Morning NPH or lente | 67% of daily total of NPH or lente |
| 8 units | Suppertime or bedtime NPH or lente | 33% of daily total of NPH or lente |
| 8 units | Morning regular | 67% of daily total |
| 4 units | Suppertime regular | 33% of daily total |

Algorithmic adjustments of the prebreakfast and presupper regular
insulin doses can be used, as determined by your health care team.

—Two-thirds of this total will be given as NPH or lente.
—One-third of this total will be given as regular.
—Divide the total number of units to be given as NPH or lente
so that two-thirds are given before breakfast and one-third is
given at suppertime.

—Divide the total number of units to be given as regular insulin so that two-thirds are given before breakfast and one-third is given at suppertime or bedtime.

—Test your blood carefully and adjust the doses as needed.

## Other facts about premeal regular and bedtime intermediate insulin programs

- Never adjust more than one insulin at a time.

- Don't make more than two adjustments without checking with your health care team unless otherwise instructed.

- Check your weight. It is very easy to gain weight using this or any form of intensive diabetes therapy. If you do gain weight, review your meal plan with your dietitian.

- Generally, snacking may be necessary with premeal regular and bedtime intermediate insulin programs at the time of the regular insulin peaks, especially if you have been active. Snacks may also be needed if your bedtime blood glucose level is less than 200 mg/dl (or whatever value you determine should be the threshold for you).

- Your insulin can lose its stability (weaken) if left out of the refrigerator for too long a period. Do not leave the insulin out of the refrigerator for more than 30 days. It is advisable to refrigerate ultralente whenever possible. (Nonrefrigeration for travel periods should not be a problem, however.)

# CONTINUOUS SUBCUTANEOUS INSULIN INFUSION TREATMENT: THE INSULIN PUMP

## Guidelines for establishing an insulin pump program

**NOTE:** These guidelines are general and are included as an example of how an insulin pump program could be set up. They are not the only way to determine an insulin pump program. Your health care team may approach the establishment of this program in another way.

**Under no circumstances should anyone use these guidelines to switch himself or herself to an insulin pump program without the guidance of a physician who is trained in diabetes treatment and/or a diabetes health care team.**

- Establish your total daily insulin dose, either by totalling your present insulin doses or calculating it based on the body weight (approximately 0.5 unit per kilogram body weight is often used).
- The basal insulin infusion dose is about 50% of this total daily dose over a 24–hour period.
- Regular insulin boluses make up the other 50% of the total daily dose of insulin. It is often divided among the boluses so that, for a blood glucose value of 100 to 150 mg/dl, the dose makes up the following percents:

| Percent of total daily dose of REGULAR INSULIN | | Percent of total daily dose of ALL INSULINS (R+I) |
|---|---|---|
| Prebreakfast: | 40% | 20% |
| Prelunch: | 30% | 15% |
| Presupper: | 30% | 15% |

Since this is an estimated dose, round up or down when fractions occur and then adjust based on actual test results.

---

### E X A M P L E

**Calculating a dose for an insulin pump program**
Your calculated total daily dose is 40 units.

#### —Your pump doses would be:

| Insulin | Given as: | Represents about: |
|---------|-----------|-------------------|
| 20 units | Total daily basal insulin | 50% of daily total insulin |
| 20 units | Total daily regular bolus doses | 50% of daily total insulin |

#### Dosage breakdown

| | | |
|---------|-----------|-------------------|
| 0.8 units/hour | Basal insulin dose (for 20 units given over 24 hours) | 100% of daily basal given over 24 hours |
| 8 units | Prebreakfast regular insulin bolus for glucose values of 100–150 mg/dl | 40% of daily total of regular |
| 6 units | Prelunch regular insulin bolus for glucose values of 100–150 mg/dl | 30% of daily total of regular |
| 6 units | Presupper regular insulin bolus for glucose values of 100–150 mg/dl | 30% of daily total of regular |

---

An algorithm is then designed by increasing the dose (usually by one unit) for every 50 points above 150 mg/dl, and decreasing for every 50 points below 100 mg/dl.

### Well day insulin adjustments of a continuous subcutaneous insulin infusion (pump) program

Before adjusting insulin, you must be:

—Following your meal plan
—Using your testing equipment correctly
—Not sick
—Sure you are not having hypoglycemic reactions and rebounding

—Sure the pump is working properly, that there are no occlusions in the infusion set, and that there is no infection or inflammation at the insertion site.

Be sure you have discussed your initial blood glucose level goals with your health care team and that they are safe and realistic. For people seeking DCCT level control, your goal inevitably will, over time and through experience, become lower than what is listed here. Generally, initial goals established to help you get underway will be:

Fasting:                            100–150 mg/dl

Premeals and bedtime:    100–150 mg/dl

However, your goals may be different. The frequency of blood glucose test results outside these limits, or the duration of time with tests out of these limits, may vary from individual to individual. Be sure you have discussed with your health care team when you should begin "well day adjustments."


## For high blood glucose levels:

*High fasting values*—After 4 days in a row of high fasting blood glucose test results (whatever your health care team defines as high for you), verify by checking a blood glucose level at 2 A.M.

—*If the 2 A.M. test result is low* (as suggested by a value under 100 mg/dl), the high fasting test result may be due to rebound. Decrease the basal insulin by 0.1 to 0.2 units per hour. Alternatively, lower the basal but initiate a higher alternate basal to run during the latter part of your sleep.

—*If the 2 A.M. test result is high* (100 mg/dl or more), the high fasting test result may be due to insufficient insulin action overnight. Increase the basal insulin rate by 0.1 to 0.2 units per hour.

—*If you already use an alternate basal rate during the night,* it may be this alternate basal that you should increase. If you have multiple alternate basal rates, consult your health care team about which one to adjust.

Wait *at least 4 days* between each change in the basal insulin infusion rate.

### For high premeal test results, adjust the sliding scale algorithm doses for regular insulin

—*For prelunch high blood sugars* (whatever parameters your health care team has determined for you), increase the morning scale by 1 unit.
—*For presupper high blood sugars* (whatever parameters your health care team has determined for you), increase the lunchtime scale by 1 unit.
—*For bedtime high blood sugars* (whatever parameters your health care team has determined for you), increase the suppertime scale by 1 unit.

Wait *two days* minimum between each adjustment in the sliding scale algorithm. Again, your goals will become stricter with practice.

### For low blood sugars:

*If your blood sugar is low* (below whatever level your health care team has set as your lower goal) for *three days in a row,* at the same time of day, without symptoms of an insulin reaction or explanations due to a temporary decrease in your eating or increase in your activity, decrease the appropriate insulin as noted above under the "high blood sugar" section.

Wait *two days* between each adjustment in your sliding scales, and four days between each adjustment in the basal insulin dose.

If you have an unexplained hypoglycemic insulin reaction (a blood glucose level under 60 mg/dl that you cannot explain by a decrease in food or an increase in activity, or an error in your insulin dose), *decrease* the appropriate insulin a the *very next day,* as noted above.

If you have an alternate basal, evaluate the time period that the alternate basal is in effect. If the hypoglycemic reaction has occurred during that period, decrease the alternate basal by 0.1 unit/hour (or as instructed by your health care team).

### Sick day guidelines for people using an insulin infusion pump

- Test your blood glucose level every 3 to 4 hours day and night. Whenever your blood glucose level is 240 mg/dl or higher, test the urine for ketones.

- Always take your insulin, even if you are unable to eat.

    —If you CAN eat, drink plenty of water or sugar-free beverages, about one cup each hour, and follow your usual meal plan.

    — If you CAN'T eat, every other hour while you are awake drink one cup of fluids with sugar, such as regular soda, popsicles, ice cream, or lemonade, alternating with fluids without sugar on opposite hours.

    —If you have nausea or are vomiting, and are unable to hold down either food or drink, call your physician immediately.
- Rest
- Drink plenty of fluids
- Additional insulin is usually recommended if the blood glucose values are at or above 240 mg/dl, especially if urine ketones are present.
- Additional insulin is determined according to the following plan:

**Basal insulin doses:**

    –Single basal: increase basal dose 50%
    –Multiple basal doses: increase each basal dose by 50%
If you are confused about how to increase your basal doses or concerned that the recommended increases may cause hypoglycemia, contact your health care team.

---

### E X A M P L E

If your basal dose is 0.8 units/hour, increase the dose to 1.2 units/hour.

50% of 0.8 = 0.4 units.      0.8 + 0.4 = 1.2 units/hour

---

### Insulin bolus increases:

Next, increase your premeal bolus. To calculate the dose of additional insulin (sick day bolus):

- Determine the total daily dose by adding the total daily basal infusion to the sum of the regular insulin boluses you would give for blood glucose values in the 100-150 mg/dl range before each meal and snack.
- Your sick day bolus is 10% if the blood glucose is 240-400 mg/dl with negative ketones.
- Your sick day bolus is 20% if the blood glucose is 240-400 mg/dl with positive ketones, or if the blood glucose level is over 400 mg/dl, regardless of the urine ketones.

---

## E X A M P L E

**Calculating sick day insulin booster**
**for an insulin pump program**

**—Your usual insulin pump doses are:**

| Insulin | Given as: |
|---|---|
| 19 units | Basal dose given over 24 hours (0.8 units/hour) |
| 8 units | Prebreakfast insulin bolus for glucose values of 100–150 mg/dl |
| 5 units | Prelunch insulin bolus for glucose values of 100–150 mg/dl |
| 5 units | Presupper insulin bolus for glucose values of 100–150 mg/dl |
| **37 units** | **Total daily insulin dose** |

**Your sick day booster doses would be:**

4 units (rounded from 3.7) regular insulin for a catch-up dose of 10% of daily total

7 units (rounded from 7.4) regular insulin for a catch-up dose of 20% of daily total

---

- Take the bolus booster every 3 to 4 hours as needed when blood glucose elevations warrant it. If it is needed at the same time as a premeal bolus, add the booster quantity to the dose of regular insulin you would have normally taken, by algorithm, for that given glucose level.

- If your blood glucose level has not come down within 4 hours, contact your health care team. Also, at this time, it may be necessary to come off the pump, and to use injected insulin. In general, before you become sick, review with your health care team the protocol you should use.
- Check your syringe often when using sick day rules. Remember, you will be taking additional insulin for a sick day, and you may need to refill the syringe more often.
- Stop using the sick day booster when your blood sugar comes down below 240 mg/dl.
- Ketones take longer to leave the body, so you may see ketones in the urine the next day. Drink extra fluids to help flush out the ketones.
- Treat the illness appropriately. If unsure, contact your physician for advice.

## Switching from an insulin pump program to a program using regular and NPH or lente

### Switching to NPH/lente but retaining the regular insulin algorithm

Calculate the total daily basal insulin dose over 24 hours and give the this total as NPH or lente, divided as follows:

A.M. dose: 60% of the total basal dose

P.M. dose: 40% of the total basal dose (before supper)

Continue to use morning and predinner sliding scale (algorithm) for regular insulin. Omit or reduce the noontime regular, as NPH will pick up at the same time.

### Switching to NPH/lente using a split mix instead of the algorithm

Calculate the total daily dose of insulin by adding up the basal doses plus the doses of regular insulin as determined by the adjustment algorithm for a blood glucose value of 100 to 150 mg/dl.

— Two-thirds of this total will be given as NPH or lente.
— One-third of this total will be given as regular.

— Divide the total number of units to be given as NPH or lente so that two-thirds are given before breakfast, and one-third are given at suppertime.

— Divide the total number of units to be given as regular insulin so that two-thirds are given before breakfast, and one-third are given at suppertime.

— Test the blood carefully and adjust the doses as needed.

## E X A M P L E

**Insulin pump program conversion to split-mix program**

**—Your usual insulin pump doses are:**

| Insulin | Given as: |
|---|---|
| 24 units | Basal dose given over 24 hours |
| 8 units | Bolus for a fasting blood glucose level of 100-150 mg/dl |
| 5 units | Bolus for a prelunch blood glucose level of 100-150 mg/dl |
| 5 units | Bolus for a presupper blood glucose level of 100-150 mg/dl |
| **42 units** | **Total daily insulin dose** |

**Split-Mix Program:**

| Insulin | Given as: | Represents about: |
|---|---|---|
| 28 units | Total daily NPH or lente | 67% of daily total insulin |
| 14 units | Total daily regular | 33% of daily total insulin |

### Dosage Breakdown

| | | |
|---|---|---|
| 19 units | Morning NPH or lente | 67% of total daily NPH or lente |
| 9 units | Suppertime or bedtime NPH or lente | 33% of total daily NPH or lente |
| 9 units | Morning regular | 67% of daily regular dose |
| 5 units | Suppertime regular | 33% of daily regular dose |

Algorithmic adjustments of the prebreakfast and presupper regular insulin doses can be used, as determined by your health care team.

## Other facts about insulin pump programs

■ Never adjust more than one change at a time, either the basal or the premeal boluses.

■ Don't make more than two adjustments without checking with your health care team unless otherwise instructed.

■ Check infusion sites frequently for signs of infection.

■ Check your weight. It is very easy to gain weight using this or any form of intensive insulin therapy. If you do gain weight, review your meal plan with your dietitian.

■ Generally, snacking is not routinely necessary with pump therapy programs. However, snacks may be needed before or after exercise, or if your bedtime blood glucose level is less than 200 mg/dl (or whatever value you determine is necessary for you).

■ Your insulin can lose its stability (weaken) if left out of the refrigerator for too long a period. Do not leave the insulin out of the refrigerator for more than 30 days. (Nonrefrigeration for travel periods should not be a problem, however.)

■ Buffered regular insulin is phosphate buffered. It will crystallize if mixed with any other type of insulin. Buffered regular insulin must be taken alone.

## Signs of infection when using insulin pump therapy

One important aspect of insulin pump therapy is to observe the insulin injection site daily for signs of infection. Be suspicious of infection if you observe any of the following signs:

–Redness            –Swelling

–Warmth            –Fever

–Pain            –Abscess formation

–Drainage. What color? Any color?

Also, if you notice changes in the appearance of the insertion site or skin around it, ask yourself the following:

—How long have I had this skin condition?

—Has it occurred previously?

—Where is the insertion site located? Are any other sites involved?

—What about the surrounding skin? (Changes in the appearance of the surrounding skin would suggest a tape allergy.)

—What is the size of the area involved? Is it confined to the insertion site only, or does it cover a larger area?

—How has this condition affected my blood glucose readings?

### Treatment for infections

- Remove the pump and reinsert it at another site, distant from the infected area, with a new infusion set.

- Cleanse the area thoroughly with soap and water.

- Apply a clear antibiotic ointment such as Bacitracin® or Neosporin®.

- Cover with a sterile dressing and paper tape.

- Take your temperature and see if you have a fever.

- Monitor blood glucose levels closely. Use sick day rules if necessary.

- Notify your health care team immediately.

# CALCULATING DAILY VOLUME FOR INSULIN PUMP THERAPY

### Establish the following:

- Basal rate

    —One basal rate:

    Hourly basal rate x 24 (hour in the day) = _____

    —Multiple basal rates:

    Rate 1 x number of hours that rate is running = _____

    Rate 2 x number of hours that rate is running = _____

    Rate 3 x number of hours that rate is running = _____

    Total basal for 24 hours = _____

- Premeal maximum dose

    —Breakfast maximum = _____

    —Lunchtime maximum = _____

    —Dinnertime maximum = _____

- Infusion set

    —42" equals 27 units of insulin = _____

    —24" equals 18 units of insulin = _____

- Priming the tubing = 20 units

- Connecting/reconnecting: approximately 5 units for each connection/reconnection = _____

**Total amount needed per day = _____**

# EXERCISE GUIDELINES

Regular exercise increases your body's sensitivity to insulin, and therefore increases effectiveness of your injected insulin. Exercise will also help lower the level of blood fats (cholesterol and triglycerides). It contributes to the fitness of your heart and blood vessels and can help you control your weight.

## General guidelines

- Make sure your diabetes is in good control.

- Do not exercise when your blood glucose level is 300 mg/dl or higher, especially when ketones are present.

- Be sure to obtain medical clearance before you begin an exercise program. If you have retinopathy, check with your ophthalmologist.

   —**Type of exercise.** The best exercise is a continuous activity that uses a large amount of energy over a period of time. Examples include brisk walking, running, bicycling, swimming, and dancing. If you use an insulin pump and are engaging in contact sports, skiing, or swimming, it is best to remove the pump.

   —**Intensity.** To get maximum benefit from exercise, you need to achieve 60 to 85% of your maximum heart rate (MHR). MHR equals 220 minus your age. This gives the maximum heart beats per minute. Multiply this amount by 0.6 and 0.85 to determine the 60 and 85% MHR goal for you. Then, based on your MHR, determine what is 60 to 85%.

   —**Duration.** If you are just getting started, begin with 10 to 20 minutes. If you are active, aim for 30 to 45 minutes of activity.

   —**Frequency.** An exercise period each day is ideal. Exercise every other day is essential if your program is to help manage your diabetes.

   —**Timing.** The best time to exercise is one to two hours after a meal, ideally the largest meal of the day.

—**Injection sites.** Choose injection sites that are less likely to be affected by the working muscles.

—**Fluids.** Water is best as it is easily absorbed.

—**Monitoring.** Because exercise works very differently from one person to the next, it is best to monitor frequently to see how that particular activity affected you. Test your blood before and, most importantly, after exercise. Also check several hours later to observe for the lag effect. In addition, it's a good idea to check your blood during exercise if you think your blood sugar is low or if you are having problem with the lag effect or rebounding.

—**Insulin adjustment.** Insulin adjustment works best when you have planned for the exercise. You will need to figure out which insulin is peaking at the time you plan to exercise and adjust accordingly. Keep records of your adjustments, so you an use them for reference later on.

Never adjust ultralente for exercise unless your health care team tells you to do so. Work with the algorithm scale. Try decreasing your algorithm scale by 1 to 2 units. If you have made an adjustment and it did not work, adjust it again the next time. Remember that premeal algorithms are not "etched in stone" and can be adjusted for variations in activity.

If you are using an insulin pump and plan to exercise all day, it may be necessary to decrease the basal only if you plan to exercise all day. You should first discuss this with your health care team.

Insulin adjustment will depend on the time of the day, the intensity of the exercise, and your past experiences.

When someone has been getting in shape for a while, frequently the overall insulin dose will decline somewhat.

—**Food adjustments.** Always carry fast acting carbohydrate! Refer to lists (Chapter 8) for specific suggestions for food adjustments.

# HYPERGLYCEMIA

**Fasting hyperglycemia**

**(Blood glucose level before breakfast is too high)**

**Possible causes:**

1. Insulin given the night before does not last long enough to maintain enough of an effect the following morning.

2. An increased need for insulin action occurs at the end of the sleep cycle—the dawn phenomenon.

3. A hypoglycemic reaction occurs during the night with resultant rebound hyperglycemia by morning—the Somogyi phenomenon.

Identify the cause by testing blood glucose levels at bedtime, during the night, and first thing in the morning on repeated occasions. Look for the following suggestive patterns:

### 1. Suggestive of insufficient insulin duration:

- Bedtime glucose level in desired range

- Middle of the night glucose level a little higher than bedtime glucose level

- Fasting glucose level too high

### 2. Suggestive of dawn phenomenon:

- Bedtime glucose level in desired range

- Middle of the night glucose level in desired range, often slightly below bedtime level, but not generally under 80 mg/dl

- Fasting glucose level too high

### 3. Suggestive of Somogyi phenomenon:

The classic blood glucose patterns:

- Bedtime glucose level in desired range
- Middle of the night glucose level low, suggested by a value often under 80 mg/dl and certainly less than 65 mg/dl
- Fasting glucose level too high

If the classic pattern does not appear, certain circumstantial evidence may indicate that nocturnal hypoglycemia has occurred. Symptoms suggestive of nocturnal hypoglycemia include:

- Nightmares
- Restless sleep
- Perspiration during the night beyond what would be expected from the room temperature
- Morning headaches
- Morning ketonuria (urine ketones)

**Note:** If the initial assumption was that morning hyperglycemia was due to insufficient insulin duration or the dawn phenomenon and appropriate adjustments for those problems did not correct the hyperglycemia or, especially, if they made it worse, consider the Somogyi phenomenon and adjust accordingly. If those adjustments correct the hyperglycemia, then the problem was, indeed, Somogyi!

**Comment:** In general, if unsure, first adjust as instructed below for the most likely explanation. Then, if the problem does not resolve, try something else. The problem could be a combination of more than one of these factors, perhaps different ones occurring on different days.

### Suggested insulin adjustments to consider

### 1. For insufficient insulin duration:

—Programs using a prebreakfast mixture of regular and intermediate insulins, regular insulin before supper, and intermediate insulin at bedtime

- Increase the bedtime dose of intermediate insulin.

- Take the bedtime dose later if possible.

- If the bedtime glucose level is high also, try either increasing the suppertime regular insulin dose or adding a small dose (2 to 3 units) of intermediate insulin mixed with the suppertime regular insulin dose (perhaps reducing the suppertime regular and bedtime intermediate initially until the effect of these changes can be assessed).

- Consider using a "true" intensive diabetes program

**—Programs using ultralente twice daily and regular before meals**

- Increase both ultralente doses equally.

- If this causes hypoglycemia at other times of the day, give more ultralente at night and less ultralente in the morning. (This is most effective if human ultralente is being used.)

- If bedtime glucose level is also slightly high, use more regular before supper.

**Note:** Ultralente is a very long-acting insulin and rarely does its action not act long enough. If you are on ultralente and experiencing fasting hyperglycemia, the problem is most likely related to the dawn phenomenon. If the above maneuvers fail, consider changing to a program that is more effective against the dawn phenomenon such as premeal regular/bedtime intermediate or a pump.

**—Programs using premeal regular and bedtime intermediate (NPH or lente) insulin**

- Give the bedtime insulin dose later.

- If your bedtime glucose level is also slightly high, use more regular before supper.

- In theory, with the human insulins, lente may act a little longer than NPH. While this difference may be more theoretical than real in many instances, if you are using NPH, it doesn't hurt to try lente.

- Consider using a pump with alternate basal rates.

—Programs using insulin pumps

The issue of insufficient duration is not usually seen with a pump because of the constant infusion. Usually, the problem would be due to the dawn phenomenon.

## 2. For the dawn phenomenon:

—Programs using a prebreakfast mixture of regular and intermediate insulins, regular insulin before supper, and intermediate insulin at bedtime.

- Increase the bedtime dose of intermediate insulin. Watch carefully for hypoglycemia earlier during the night, however.
- Take the bedtime dose later if possible.
- Consider using a "true" intensive diabetes program.

—Programs using ultralente twice daily and regular before meals

- Increase both ultralente doses equally.
- If these increases cause hypoglycemia at other times of the day, give more ultralente at night and less in the morning. (This is most effective if human ultralente is being used.)
- Some people have tried using intermediate (NPH or lente) insulin at night, either mixed with the regular and ultralente at suppertime or as an additional injection at bedtime. However, doing this may cause much confusion as to which insulin is affecting the blood glucose levels at what time. In general, we do not encourage this approach, but it is not incorrect or harmful if you are fortunate enough to be able to sort out the effects of the various insulins. This approach is not recommended except under supervision of a health care team skilled in intensive insulin treatment programs.
- Consider changing to a program that is more effective against the dawn phenomenon.

- Premeal regular/bedtime intermediate is the most effective MDI program when dawn phenomenon is the problem.
- Insulin infusion pumps, with the ability to use alternate basal doses, are more effective than any of the MDI programs in controlling the dawn phenomenon.

## —Programs using premeal regular and bedtime intermediate (NPH or lente) insulin

- Increase the bedtime dose of intermediate insulin but watch carefully for hypoglycemia earlier during the night.
- If the bedtime glucose level is also slightly high, use more regular before supper.
- Consider using a pump. Insulin infusion pumps, with the ability to use alternate basal doses, are more effective than any of the MDI programs in controlling the dawn phenomenon.

## —Programs using insulin pumps

- If you have a single basal rate all day and night, you could increase the basal rate. You might need to concurrently reduce the bolus dose quantities to prevent hypoglycemia during the day.
- Try using an alternate basal dose during the night with a higher basal infusion rate. Guidelines for starting this alternate basal include:
  - Start the alternate basal somewhere between 1 A.M. and 3 A.M.
  - Run the alternate basal until about 6 or 7 A.M.
  - Start with an alternate basal dose that is only slightly higher than the previous insulin dose, and then work that alternate basal dose upward gradually and stepwise, as needed.
- If you are already using an alternate basal dose during the night:
  - Increase the infusion rate of that alternate basal dose.
  - Start the alternate (higher) basal earlier during the night.

**3. Failure to correct fasting hyperglycemia when you have assumed that the cause was either insufficient insulin duration or the dawn phenomenon. This may occur if the real cause was undetected Somogyi phenomenon.**

- Adjustments that have been made will either not correct the problem or make it worse.

- After the fasting hyperglycemia, the next blood glucose levels may actually come back into target levels quite well because:

    • Hyperglycemia due to rebound tends to correct itself easier and faster than hyperglycemia due to insufficient insulin quantity.

    • The algorithm for more regular insulin or even the overall insulin dose acting overnight may have been inadvertently designed to provide enough insulin to compensate for the rebound hyperglycemia.

- If you suspect any of the above, go on to adjustments listed below for the Somogyi phenomenon.

**4. Somogyi phenomenon:**

**—Programs using a prebreakfast mixture of regular and intermediate insulins, regular insulin before supper, and intermediate insulin at bedtime**

• Decrease the bedtime dose of intermediate insulin.

• If the bedtime glucose level is also low, consider reducing the suppertime regular insulin dose as well.

• Consider taking (or increasing) a bedtime snack.

• Consider using a "true" intensive diabetes program.

**—Programs using ultralente twice daily and regular before meals**

• Reduce the two ultralente doses equally.

- Reduce the suppertime ultralente dose, leaving the morning dose alone. This is especially effective if human ultralente is being used or if the suppertime ultralente dose is already larger than the morning dose.

- Consider premeal regular and bedtime intermediate if the bedtime dose can be given late enough to ensure that it peaks at dawn and not earlier during the night.

- Consider a pump with alternate basals if the approaches listed above do not work.

## —Programs using premeal regular and bedtime intermediate (NPH or lente) insulin

- Decrease the bedtime dose of intermediate insulin.

- If your bedtime glucose level is also slightly low, use less regular before supper, so that you will not be heading downward too rapidly when the bedtime intermediate insulin begins working.

- Consider using a pump with alternate basal rates.

## —Programs using insulin pumps

- With a single basal rate all day and night, you could decrease the basal rate. You might need to concurrently increase the bolus dose quantities to prevent hyperglycemia during the day.

- Use an alternate basal dose during the late evening and early nighttime, with a lower basal infusion rate. Some people doing this also need a third basal later during the night, because with the reduction of the early night basal, fasting hyperglycemia is seen due to the dawn phenomenon.

- If already on an alternate basal dose during the night:
  - Decrease the quantity of the basal rate that acts during the period immediately preceding the time of the hypoglycemia.
  - Start the alternate basal dose that acts during the period immediately preceding the time of the hypoglycemia earlier during the night.

For all programs, if the Somogyi phenomenon had been causing upward momentum in the blood glucose levels at the time of the fasting insulin dose, it is possible that the quantity of insulin given at that time had been adjusted to compensate for this upward movement. Once the Somogyi phenomenon has been eliminated, you may find that less insulin is needed first thing in the morning.

### For all intensive diabetes programs and for all problems

—Examine evening eating habits to be sure that the quantity of the food or the types of food are not the cause of the problem.

- Too much rapid-acting carbohydrate or not enough complex carbohydrate, protein, or fat may cause an early nighttime rise that doesn't persist through the night and could cause the Somogyi phenomenon.

- Too much food might cause too much of a rise through the night.

—Examine the activity pattern to rule out the lag effect (hypoglycemia hours after activity).

## Blood glucose too high before lunch, supper or at bedtime

## Possible causes:

1. Not enough insulin action during the preceding time interval.

2. Blood glucose level was too high going into that time interval. For example, for high sugar at suppertime, it was also too high at lunchtime. The insulin action during that time (in this example, between lunch and supper) could not bring the glucose down.

3. Improper meal plan design/noncompliance for the previous meal.

4. Hypoglycemic reactions during the previous interval with resultant rebound.

5. Insufficient duration of action of the insulin acting over that previous interval.

Identify the cause by testing blood glucose levels at the appropriate times before meals or bedtime, 1 or 2 hours after meals, with activity, and with symptoms suggestive of hypoglycemia.

## 1. Signs suggestive of not enough insulin action during the preceding time interval would be:

- Glucose before the previous meal in target range

- Glucose after the previous meal at or above target range

- Glucose at the time in question (premeal or bedtime) above target range

## 2. Signs suggestive of high sugar from before the previous meal persisting:

- Glucose before the previous meal above target range

- Glucose after the previous meal above target range

- Glucose at the time in question (premeal or bedtime) above target range

## 3. Signs suggestive of improper meal plan design or compliance:

- Glucose before the previous meal in the target range

- Glucose after the previous meal well above target range

- Glucose at the time in question (premeal or bedtime) above target range

- Review of meal plan shows that you have not been following it or that it contains too much quantity, too much rapid acting carbohydrate, or not enough protein, fat, or fiber

### 4. Signs suggestive of hypoglycemic reactions with resultant rebounds:

- Glucose before the previous meal in the target range

- Glucose after the previous meal below target range, either at 1 or 2 hours after the meal, or at some other time

- Symptoms during that interval suggestive of hypoglycemia

- Glucose at the time in question (premeal or bedtime) above target range

- Review of meal plan shows that you have not been following it and eating less, or that it does not contain enough carbohydrates, or both

- Review of activity shows an increased amount

### 5. Signs suggestive of insufficient insulin duration:

- Glucose before the previous meal in the target range

- Glucose 1 or 2 hours after the previous meal in the target range

- Glucose at some other time after the meal beginning to rise

- Glucose at the time in question (premeal or bedtime) above target range

## Suggested insulin adjustments to consider

### 1. Not enough insulin during the previous interval:

- Increase the regular insulin dose before the previous meal

  1. If this does not solve the problem and there is no problem with hypoglycemia:
     - Increase the regular insulin dose further
     - Adjust the diet: reduce calories and/or adjust composition of the diet

2. If this does not solve the problem and there is a problem with hypoglycemia during that interval:

   - Decrease the regular insulin dose and increase the longer acting insulin acting during that time period: the ultralente or the pump basal. (This is not possible with premeal regular and bedtime intermediate. If this program is being used, see instructions for insufficient duration on page 223.)
   - Adjust the diet for more carbohydrate.

## 2. High sugar from before the previous meal persisting:

—Adjust the insulin during that previous interval to correct that sugar level.

—Increase the algorithm for regular insulin before that previous meal so that it is more effective at bringing a glucose level that starts off too high back down into the target range.

## 3. Improper meal plan design or compliance:

—Follow the meal plan better!

—Review your meal plan with the dietitian to adjust the quantity of food and/or food composition.

## 4. Hypoglycemic reactions with resultant rebounds:

—Review your meal and activity plan to be sure that these are properly balanced.

—**Programs using a prebreakfast mixture of regular and intermediate insulins, regular insulin before supper, and intermediate insulin at bedtime.**

   • Reduce the quantity of insulin covering that time period.

- Beware of "crossover periods," particularly prelunch, where both the end of the effect from the morning regular, and the beginning of the effect from the morning intermediate insulins are both possible contributors.

## —Programs using ultralente and premeal regular

- Reduce the quantity of regular insulin given before the previous meal. Eliminate hypoglycemic reactions and see if the glucose levels before the next meal come in on target.

- If reducing the regular insulin dose alone does not solve the problem, also reduce the dose of ultralente acting at that time. You may need to increase the regular insulin dose again if you do this.

- If reducing the regular and the ultralente does not solve the problem, and if diet and activity have been examined and adjusted as much as is possible, consider using a program with premeal regular insulin and bedtime intermediate insulin. Such a program may allow enough of a drop in the insulin level to prevent hypoglycemia.

## —Programs using premeal regular insulin and bedtime intermediate insulin

- Reduce the dose of regular insulin given before the previous meal. Eliminate hypoglycemic reactions and see if the glucose levels before the next meal come in on target.

## —Programs using insulin pumps

- Reduce the bolus of regular insulin given before the previous meal. Eliminate hypoglycemic reactions and see if the glucose levels before the next meal come in on target.

- If reducing the bolus of regular insulin alone does not solve the problem, reduce also the basal insulin dose acting at that time. If doing so causes a high glucose level at some other time, either adjust the bolus covering that time, or consider an alternate basal dose.

## 5. Insufficient duration of action of the insulin acting over that previous interval:

—Programs using a prebreakfast mixture of regular and intermediate insulins, regular insulin before supper, and intermediate insulin at bedtime

- If this occurs during the morning, affecting the prelunch glucose level, increase the morning intermediate insulin.

- If this occurs during the afternoon, affecting the presupper glucose level, consider:

  - Increasing the morning intermediate insulin dose, provided prelunch hypoglycemia does not occur (a snack could prevent this latter problem)

  - Consider using a premeal regular and bedtime intermediate insulin program, so that the control of the afternoon and presupper glucose levels could be managed by prelunch regular insulin. (Occasionally, also using a small dose of ultralente mixed with the morning regular dose can help as the daytime intervals are particularly long.)

—Programs using ultralente and regular

- It is likely that it is the regular insulin that is running out. Increase the ultralente insulin dose acting over that time period. Beware: doing so may necessitate reduction of the regular insulin dose acting at that time, or some other time.

—Programs using premeal regular insulin and bedtime intermediate

- With no basal effect in this program, if the regular insulin does not last long enough, consider adding another type of insulin to help bridge this time span.

  - Intermediate insulin can help span longer lengths of time between meals, but often with some carryover into the next time span. This may require a downward adjustment of the regular insulin that covers that interval.

- A small dose of ultralente can provide better basal coverage, but will carry over much longer. Ultralente is useful if there is a very long stretch of time from breakfast, through lunch, and up to dinner.

- Consider changing to another program that will help bridge these longer time spans such as the ultralente program or a pump.

—Programs using insulin pumps

- Decrease the regular insulin and increase the basal insulin dose acting over that time period. If doing so causes hypoglycemia at some other time, use an alternate basal to span that time period.

## Blood glucose level too high one to two hours after meals, but on target before meals

### Possible causes:

1. Not quite enough insulin action during the preceding time interval. This insulin action is just enough to hold the premeal glucose level on target. However, there is not enough insulin available, either from the previous time period or from that meal's prandial insulin injection, to prevent postprandial hyperglycemia when the food gets to the bloodstream.

2. Improper meal plan design/noncompliance for the previous meal.

3. Hypoglycemic reactions during the previous interval with resultant rebound.

Identify the cause by testing blood glucose levels at appropriate times before meals or bedtime, 1 to 2 hours after meals, with activity, and with symptoms suggestive of hypoglycemia.

**1. Signs suggestive of not quite enough insulin action during the preceding time interval would be:**

–Glucose before the previous meal is in the targeted range

–Glucose after the previous meal is above the targeted range

–Glucose before the next meal is on target

–Meal plan is proper and being followed

**2. Signs suggestive of improper meal plan design or noncompliance for the previous meal:**

–Pattern as in number 1 above

–Meal plan contains too much concentrated carbohydrate or not enough protein, fat, or fiber

**3. Signs suggestive of hypoglycemic reactions during the previous interval, with resultant rebound:**

Pattern as in number 1 above but also with evidence of hypoglycemia based on at least one of the following:

- Symptoms of hypoglycemia
- A low blood glucose reading during the previous interval.
- Patterns showing a dip in the glucose level during the previous interval but without symptoms of hypoglycemia or documentation of a low glucose level in the absence of any other explanation for the subsequent hyperglycemia.

## Suggested adjustments to consider

### 1. For not enough insulin during the previous interval:

—If regular insulin has been acting over that interval, increase the dose, but beware of hypoglycemia.

—If the previous period is overnight, increase the overnight insulin or pump basal, but beware of hypoglycemia.

—If combination insulin is acting over the previous period (regular plus pump basal or ultralente) and increasing the regular causes hypoglycemia, try increasing the basal or ultralente dose.

### 2. For improper meal plan:

—If you have not followed a meal plan that is correctly designed, begin to do so!

—If you have been following the plan, consult your dietitian to adjust it to include more protein, fiber, or fat.

### 3. Hypoglycemic reactions during the previous interval with resultant rebound hyperglycemia:

—Follow the instructions listed in the previous section for adjusting for hypoglycemia.

# HYPOGLYCEMIA

## Treatment of hypoglycemic reactions

**If you are conscious and able to eat:**

—Check your blood sugar. If low, proceed to next item.

—Eat a rapid-acting carbohydrate source (see Appendix 9).

—Wait 15 minutes; check blood sugar again.

—If blood sugar is below 70 mg/dl, re-treat with rapid-acting carbohydrate.

—If blood sugar is above 70 mg/dl, but your next meal is more than 1 hour away, eat one bread exchange with at least 2 protein exchanges.

**If you are not conscious or unable to eat, people around you should:**

—Not force you to try to eat or drink

—Someone should be trained to administer glucagon so he or she can do so if needed.

- If you do regain consciousness within 5 to 10 minutes, be sure to eat some food as instructed by your health care team.

- If you do not regain consciousness after 5 to 10 minutes, you should be given a second injection of glucagon. If you then awaken, eat as instructed.

- If you do not regain consciousness within 5 to 10 minutes or after the second injection of glucagon, an ambulance should be called and you should be transported to the nearest emergency room for intravenous glucose treatment.

**NOTE:** If there is any question that your changed level of consciousness may be due to anything other than simply a low blood glucose level (such as after an injury or after having headaches, chest pain, severe shortness of breath, or abdominal pain), you should be brought to an emergency room whether or not glucagon is tried or is successful.

- If no one near you knows how to administer glucagon, an ambulance should be called and you should be transported to the nearest emergency room for treatment.

Once the hypoglycemia has been corrected, try to determine whether the reaction was "explained" (you could identify the reason for the reaction) or "unexplained" (you could not identify an explanation for the reaction).

## Possible reasons for "explained" reactions include:

1. Not enough food.
2. Delayed food.
3. Insufficient or missed snacks.
4. Too much activity without increased food or decreased insulin.

   –A one-time increase in activity.

   –Generally increased activity over a few days or weeks.
5. Too much insulin.
6. Alcohol
7. A combination of the above.

### If the reaction was "explained," then you should:

— Try to prevent the events that precipitated the reaction from occurring again.

— Determine, either by yourself or with help from your health care team, how to compensate for the events, should they occur again, by adjusting other treatment factors such as decreased insulin or increased food.

If the reaction was "unexplained," examine your program and test results for evidence of dips in the glucose levels on other days. If you see a pattern, or if the reaction was so severe that, in the interest of safety, an immediate adjustment in insulin is indicated, use the instructions that follow.

## The approach to adjusting intensive diabetes programs due to unexplained hypoglycemic reactions:

### Nocturnal hypoglycemia (the Somogyi phenomenon)

Reactions during the night may be detected by symptoms, such as restless sleep, nightmares, etc., by awakening intentionally and testing the blood glucose level, or by suggestive evidence in glucose patterns. First check your blood sugars during the night and fasting to document glycemic patterns.

### —For all programs, examine diet and exercise

• Examine the evening eating habits to be sure that the quantity of food or the types of food are not the cause of the problem. Too much rapid-acting carbohydrate and/or not enough complex carbohydrate, protein, or fat may cause an early nighttime rise that doesn't persist through the night and could cause the Somogyi phenomenon.

• Examine the activity pattern the day before. Activity performed in the evening may result in nocturnal hypoglycemia due to the lag effect (hypoglycemia hours after activity). Remember, also, that the lag effect may persist for a number of hours, so think about activity performed earlier in the day as well.

### —Insulin adjustment for programs using a prebreakfast mixture of regular and intermediate insulin, regular insulin before supper, and intermediate insulin at bedtime.

• Decrease the bedtime dose of intermediate insulin.

- If bedtime glucose level is also slightly low, use less regular before supper, so that you will not be heading downward too rapidly when the bedtime intermediate insulin begins working.

- Consider using an ultralente program or a pump with alternate basal rates.

**—Insulin adjustments for programs using ultralente twice daily and regular before meals**

- Reduce the two ultralente doses equally.

- Reduce the suppertime ultralente dose, leaving the morning dose alone. This is especially effective if human ultralente is being used and/or if the suppertime ultralente dose is already larger than the morning dose.

- Consider the premeal regular and bedtime intermediate program if the bedtime dose can be given late enough to ensure that it peaks at dawn and not earlier during the night.

- Consider a pump with alternate basal doses if the above listed adjustments do not prevent nocturnal hypoglycemia.

**—Insulin adjustments for programs using premeal regular and bedtime intermediate (NPH or lente) insulin**

- Check the adequacy of snack at bedtime.

- Decrease the bedtime dose of intermediate insulin.

- If the bedtime glucose level is also slightly low, use less regular before supper, so you will not be heading downward too rapidly when the bedtime intermediate insulin begins working.

- Consider using a pump with alternate basal rates.

**—Insulin dose adjustments for insulin pump programs**

- With a single basal rate all day and night, you could decrease the basal rate. You might need to concurrently increase the bolus dose to prevent hyperglycemia during the day.

• Use an alternate basal dose during the late evening and early nighttime with a lower basal infusion rate. Some people doing this also need a third basal later during the night, because with the reduction of the early night basal, fasting hyperglycemia is seen due to the dawn phenomenon.

• If already on an alternate basal dose during the night:

 - Decrease the quantity of the basal rate that acts during the period immediately preceding the time of the hypoglycemia.

 - If the alternate basal dose that acts during the period immediately preceding the time of the hypoglycemia is lower than the rate before or after it, start it earlier during the night. This will allow the lower basal rate to act over a longer period of time prior to the time that hypoglycemia is likely to occur.

## Reactions during the day

### —For all programs, examine the diet and exercise

• Make sure that the quantity of food or the types of food are not the cause of the problem. Too much rapid-acting carbohydrate and/or not enough complex carbohydrate, protein, or fat may cause the glucose level to rise right after a meal, but the rise may not persist over the full time period to the next mealtime.

• If reactions occur during or just after exercise:

 - Adjust the pre-exercise snack:

  1. Increase the quantity

  2. Include more longer acting foods in the snack such as complex carbohydrate and protein

- Adjust the insulin program (see specific insulin programs listed below for details). Do you need separate exercise and nonexercise algorithm scales?

- Examine the activity pattern over the previous few hours (not just right after activity), and look for possible activity-induced hypoglycemia due to the lag effect. If present:

1. Reduce the insulin acting over the period following exercise

2. Increase the food consumed after exercise

- Take foods before and after exercise that would provide a longer acting hyperglycemic effect such as complex carbohydrates and protein, and increased fat and/or fiber

### Insulin adjustments for specific programs:

**—Insulin adjustments for programs using a prebreakfast mixture of regular and intermediate insulin, regular insulin before supper, and intermediate insulin at bedtime**

• Reduce the quantity of insulin covering that time period

• Review exercise effects

• Beware of "crossover periods," particularly prelunch, where both the end of the effect from the morning regular, and the beginning of the effect from the morning intermediate insulin are both possible contributors.

Once the above changes are made, if the glucose levels before the next meal are too high, increase the regular insulin dose again and either shorten the interval between the injection and the meal, adjust the content of the meal to contain longer acting sources of carbohydrate and other foods, or take a snack (or increase the size of the snack) between meals.

## —Programs using ultralente and premeal regular

- Reduce the quantity of regular insulin given before the previous meal to eliminate hypoglycemic reactions. Make sure the glucose levels before the next meal still are within the targeted range.

- If reducing the regular insulin dose alone does not eliminate the reactions, reduce also the dose of ultralente acting at that time. You may need to increase the regular insulin dose again if you do this. You may also need to increase the regular insulin dose at another time that is being covered by the ultralente insulin to compensate for the dose reaction.

If reducing the regular and the ultralente prevent reactions but the glucose levels before the next meal are now too high, increase the dose of regular insulin, but also increase the food consumed either at that meal or as a snack between meals.

If reducing the regular and the ultralente does not prevent reactions, and if diet and activity have been examined and adjusted as much as is possible, consider using a program with premeal regular insulin and bedtime intermediate insulin, or a pump. Such a program may allow enough of a drop in the insulin level to prevent hypoglycemia.

## —Programs using premeal regular insulin and bedtime intermediate insulin

- Reduce the dose of regular insulin given before the previous meal to eliminate hypoglycemic reactions.

*If the glucose levels before the next meal are still on target, you are all set.*

If the glucose levels before the next meal are too high, increase the regular insulin dose again and either shorten the interval between the injection and the meal, adjust the content of the meal to contain longer acting sources of carbohydrate and other foods, or take a snack (or increase the size of the snack) between meals.

- Review the exercise program.

- Are you snacking properly before (or after) exercise?

This program is, theoretically, the best of the MDI programs for exercise when hypoglycemia is a concern because you can adjust the timing of the exercise to occur when the insulin level has dropped to a low point if necessary. Consider adjusting your exercise time to occur when a regular insulin dose's action is waning.

### —Programs using an insulin pump

- Reduce the bolus of regular insulin given before the previous meal. Eliminate hypoglycemic reactions and see if the glucose levels before the next meal come in on target.

- If reducing the bolus of regular insulin alone does not prevent the reactions, or if reducing the dose further would lead to hyperglycemia before the next meal (or bedtime), reduce the basal insulin dose acting at that time. If doing so causes a high glucose level at some other time, either adjust the bolus covering that time, or consider an alternate basal dose.

- If adjusting the basal and/or bolus does not reach the proper balance:

   - Adjust the interval between the bolus and the meal (increase to further lower the subsequent glucose levels, decrease the interval to raise them)

   - Adjust the content of the meal to contain longer acting sources of carbohydrate and other foods

   - Eat a snack (or eat a bigger snack) between meals

   - Review the exercise program

   - Make sure you are snacking properly

   - Consider removing the pump during exercise

# PRODUCTS AND FOODS FOR TREATING HYPOGLYCEMIC REACTIONS

## Products

3 B-D™ glucose tablets
1/2 tube Glutose™ (80-gram container)
1/2 tube Insta-Glucose™ (31-gram container)
1 1/2 packages of Monojel™
4 Dex-4® tabs

## Foods

4 ounces of orange juice
5 to 6 ounces of regular (nondiet) soft drinks
3 to 4 teaspoons of sugar dissolved in water
8 Lifesavers™ or gummy Lifesavers™
1 tablespoon of concentrated syrup as Karo™, Coke™,
  or honey
1 small tube of cake icing
3 large marshmallows
1 tablespoon of marshmallow creme
4 teaspoons of maple syrup
6 jelly beans
9 small gumdrops
2 tablespoons of raisins
1 1/2 portions of dried fruit (actual size varies with fruit)
3 ounces of cranberry juice, regular
3 ounces of grape juice, sweetened
4 ounces of sweetened orange drink (such as Tang™, Hi-C™)
10 ounces of nonfat or low-fat milk

## Additional guidelines

— Optimal treatment of hypoglycemic reactions based on recommendations from the DCCT study:

• If the blood glucose level is between 55 and 65 mg/dl, take 3 B-D glucose tablets (15 to 20 grams fast-acting carbohydrate). Wait 15 minutes. If blood glucose is still low, repeat the same treatment.

• If blood glucose is below 55 mg/dl, take 4 B-D glucose tablets. Wait 15 minutes and repeat if the glucose is still low.

— If the recommended foods do not treat the hypoglycemia effectively, increased amounts of food or products should be tried.

— After symptoms of low blood sugar have subsided with treatment, you might need to eat something else if a meal or snack is not scheduled with the next hour. This would be necessary to prevent further hypoglycemic reactions if you anticipate a significant lag effect from prolonged exercise. In such an instance, foods providing a longer-acting carbohydrate source are recommended such as crackers and cheese or peanut butter or milk and crackers.

— Never try to give food by mouth to a person who is unconscious, nearly unconscious, or delirious. A person with these conditions caused by low blood glucose levels should be treated with glucagon injections or brought to an emergency facility.

— If in doubt or if the blood glucose level does not rise with treatment, contact a physician or emergency facility at once.

Adapted from: Krall LP, Beaser RS *Joslin Diabetes Manual,* 12th Edition. Philadelphia, Lea & Febiger, 1989, p. 252.

# SAMPLE RECORDS FOR INTENSIVE DIABETES THERAPY

Keeping proper records is a very important part of intensive diabetes therapy. Writing down why you made certain adjustments can help you build your management skills.

For monitoring records, list all test results for a given testing time in a column, so you can scan up and down for trends at that time over several days. You can also scan across the row to review glucose variations during that day. To the right of the day's blood glucose test results, list the insulin doses. (Doses can be placed along with the test results, but this is not as easy to scan.) In the far right column, leave space for comments.

Avoid record logs that list all the glucose test results in a single column in the order you obtain them. This type of log makes it more difficult to identify trends for a particular time of day.

It is helpful to quantitate variation for a "normal" day. Estimate how much activity and food is normal, then indicate variations by noting "-2" for much less, "-1 " for a little less, "+1" for a little more, and "+2" for a lot more.

The sample record on the next pages is one used by the Joslin Diabetes Center.

### Sample Record

| | Glucose Test Results | | | | | | | | |
|---|---|---|---|---|---|---|---|---|---|
| **Date** | **Breakfast** | | **Noon meal** | | **Supper** | | **Bed-time** | **Middle of night** | **Other** |
| | Before | After | Before | After | Before | After | | | |
| | | | | | | | | | |
| | | | | | | | | | |
| | | | | | | | | | |
| | | | | | | | | | |
| | | | | | | | | | |
| | | | | | | | | | |
| | | | | | | | | | |

KEY:  Regular = Regular or clear insulin
Inter. = Intermediate insulins: NPH or lente
Long = Long-acting insulins: ultralente

| Insulin | | | | | | | Comments |
|---|---|---|---|---|---|---|---|
| Before breakfast | | Before lunch | Before supper | | Bedtime | | (Food, activity, timing, etc.) |
| Regular | Long or Inter. | Regular | Regular | Long or Inter. | Regular | Long or Inter. | |
| | | | | | | | |
| | | | | | | | |
| | | | | | | | |
| | | | | | | | |
| | | | | | | | |
| | | | | | | | |
| | | | | | | | |

# JOSLIN DIABETES CENTER AND ITS AFFILIATES

For help in establishing an intensive diabetes program, or for more information on diabetes, contact any of these facilities:

Joslin Diabetes Center
One Joslin Place
Boston, MA 02215
(617) 732-2440

Joslin Center for Diabetes
Methodist Hospital of Indiana and Endocrinology Associates
1701 North Senate Boulevard
Indianapolis, IN 46206
(317) 924-8866

Joslin Center for Diabetes
St. Barnabas Medical Center
101 Old Short Hills Road
West Orange, NJ 07052
(203) 325-6555

Joslin Center for Diabetes
West Penn Hospital
5140 Liberty Avenue
Pittsburgh, PA 15224
(412) 578-1724

Joslin Center for Diabetes
Morton Plant Hospital
323 Jeffords Street
Clearwater, FL 34616
(813) 461-8300

Joslin Center for Diabetes
Baptist Hospital of Miami
8900 North Kendall Drive
Miami, FL 33176
(305) 270-3696

Nalle Clinic Diabetes Center, an Affiliate of Joslin Diabetes Center
1350 South Kings Drive
Charlotte, NC 28207
(704) 342-8110

Joslin Center for Diabetes
MacNeal Hospital
3249 South Oak Park Avenue
Berwyn, IL 60402
(708) 430-0730

Joslin Center for Diabetes
St. Luke's-Roosevelt Hospital Center
425 West 59th Street, Suite 9C
New York, NY 10019
(212) 523-8353

Joslin Center for Diabetes at Wills and Jefferson
211 South Ninth Street, Suite 600
Philadelphia, PA 19107
(215) 928-3400

**Other Resources**

American Diabetes Association
National Center
1660 Duke Street
Alexandria, VA 22314
(800) 232-3472

Juvenile Diabetes Foundation
  International
432 Park Avenue South
New York, NY 10016
(800) 223-1138

Printed in the USA
CPSIA information can be obtained
at www.ICGtesting.com
JSHW08215814O824
68134JS00014B/297